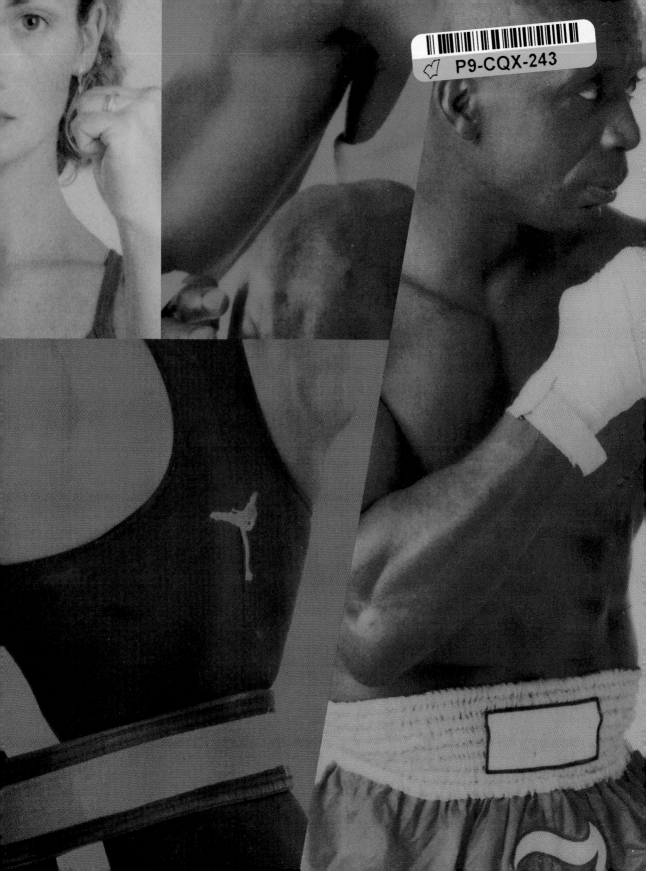

the Tae-Bo way

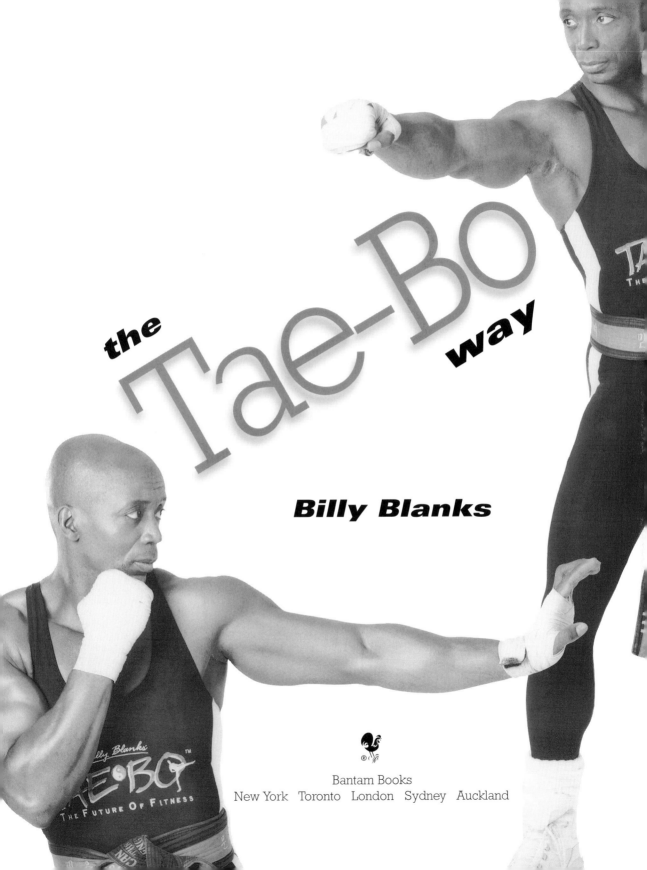

the **Tae-Bo** way

Billy Blanks

Bantam Books
New York   Toronto   London   Sydney   Auckland

Before beginning any new exercise program, including the training discussed in this book, readers are encouraged to consult with a physician to make sure it is appropriate for each individual's circumstances. The reader should follow all instructions carefully and be aware that Tae-Bo could involve physical risk, even though every effort has been made in the preparation of this book to stress the need for safety consciousness and proper technique. The author and publisher disclaim liability for any adverse effects that may result from the use or application of the information contained in this book.

The Tae-Bo Way

A Bantam Book / October 1999
All rights reserved.
Copyright © 1999 by Billy Blanks.

Book design by Amanda Kavanagh, ARK Design, NY.
Endpaper and interior photographs by RAZ / JoBee.
Illustrations by Wendy Wray.

Tae-Bo® is a registered trademark and service mark of BG Star Productions, Inc., Encino, California.

Library of Congress Cataloging-in-Publication Data

Blanks, Billy.
    The Tae-Bo way / Billy Blanks.
      p.   cm.
    ISBN 0-553-80100-7
    1. Exercise. 2. Tae-Bo (Trademark) I. Title.
  GV481.B49 1999
  613.7´1—dc21   99-42801
                  CIP

Published simultaneously in the United States and Canada

Bantam Books are published by Bantam Books, a division of Random House, Inc. Its trademark, consisting of the words "Bantam Books" and the portrayal of a rooster, is Registered in U.S. Patent and Trademark Office and in other countries. Marca Registrada. Bantam Books, 1540 Broadway, New York, New York 10036.

PRINTED IN THE UNITED STATES OF AMERICA
RRC   10 9 8 7 6 5 4 3 2 1

Do not lie to one another, since you have put off the old man with his deeds and have put on the new man, who is renewed in knowledge according to the image of Him who created him.

—Colossians 3:9–10

And do not be conformed to this world, but be transformed by the renewing of your mind, that you may prove what is that good and acceptable and perfect will of God.

—Romans 12:2

To my beloved mother and father, Mabeline and Isaac Blanks

Mom and Dad, it has always been my heart's desire to do well in my life to make you proud of the man I've become. I wasn't able to do the things for you both that I had hoped to while you were still here. But I believe you are looking at me now and smiling. I thank God you were my parents. We had so little, but you gave me so very much.

Dad: There were seventeen of us in all, but you never gave up, you never turned your back, and you never left. As a man, you were an incredible role model. You instilled in me a strong work ethic that has enabled me to reach my goals in life. You also taught me how to be a decent man with integrity. Thank you, Dad, I love you.

Mom: You were so amazing to me, and I love you so much. Thank you for showing me how to love people without prejudice, which is a beautiful gift. Your unwavering faith and love of God enabled you to always be filled with peace and joy, regardless of the circumstances. I have always admired that, and now I am at a place in my life where I really understand it.

The Lord is good and his mercy endures forever, every day, every hour, every minute, every second, all the time.

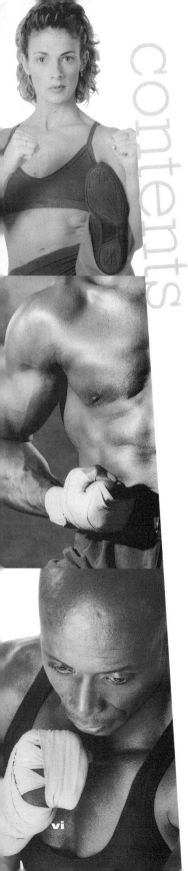

contents

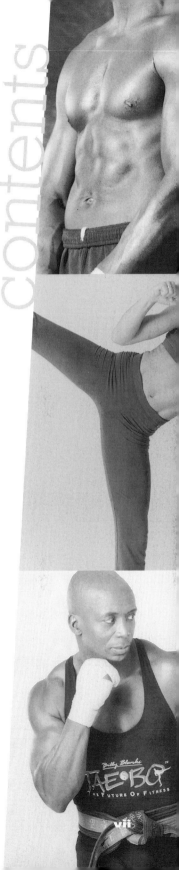

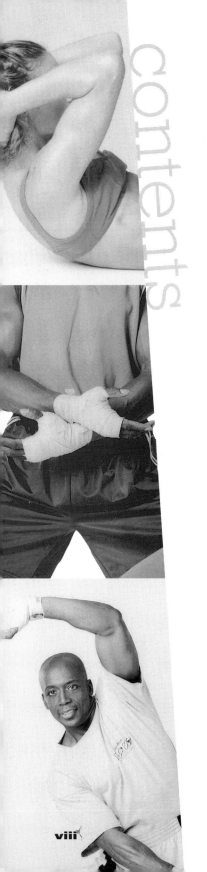

8
TROUBLESHOOTING YOUR TECHNIQUE

9
MASTERING YOUR TAE-BO WORKOUT

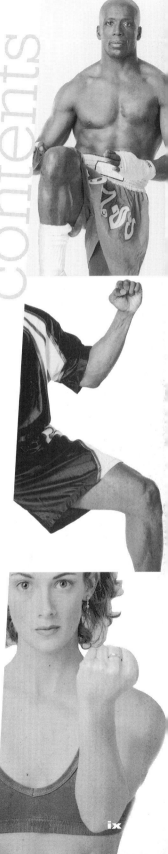

contents

An Important Message from Billy Blanks

As you may already know—and as you'll discover throughout *The Tae-Bo Way*—I designed Tae-Bo to be more than just an exercise program. I created it to challenge not only your body but your mind, your spirit, and your will. It's my hope that you will discover in Tae-Bo a force for positive change in your life. To do that, you need to exercise your self-awareness and your common sense too.

This book will tell you everything you need to know about Tae-Bo. Don't skip a word or a picture. Always remember: You are your own coach. Knowing when to slow down, modify your workout, or stop can be more important than knowing when to push ahead. Only you can know your level of fitness, your physical ability, and your health history. Only you can make that call.

I appreciate the enthusiasm and commitment students bring to Tae-Bo. The desire to move ahead, to challenge yourself, and to achieve what you never before thought possible is what makes us human. But don't forget that your first responsibility is not to work out but to work out smartly and safely. In the rush to master the next Workout, execute a higher kick, or deliver three more sets of punches, don't forget that learning to do Tae-Bo correctly takes knowledge, practice, patience, and time. Only you know when you're working out at a level that's challenging yet comfortable for you. Only you know which movements and techniques you need to modify, slow down, or devote more practice time to. Only you know how your body feels. So give your body and your Workout the attention and respect they deserve.

No matter what your age or current fitness level, I strongly recommend that you discuss Tae-Bo—or any exercise program—with your doctor especially if:

- you have not followed a regular exercise program in the past three to six months
- you are overweight or underweight for your height and build
- you lead a sedentary lifestyle with little or no regular activity (walking, riding a bicycle, etc.)
- you have a disease or chronic health problem (including but not limited to heart disease, diabetes, arthritis, high blood pressure, autoimmune disorders, etc.)
- you regularly take prescription or over-the-counter medicines (some of these may affect your ability to work out)
- you have ever suffered a sports- or exercise-related injury or any other kind of injury that might affect or be affected by exercise
- you are pregnant or soon plan to be
- you have in the past experienced unexplained incidents of dizziness, lightheadedness, or fainting
- you have any questions about whether an exercise program is right for you

Once you start doing Tae-Bo, always:

- start from the beginning and be ready to learn, even if you've been working out for years. Look, read, and be sure you fully understand each new movement and technique before you try it. Don't skip over anything here. It's all information you need to know.

◻ be realistic about what you're trying to achieve in your Workout. You may never kick as high as I do in these pictures, and that's okay. The good news is that even if your kick never rises above knee level, as long as you exercise at a good level of intensity and follow good form in your movements, you will get the same benefits from the Workout.

◻ take your time. As you're learning a new movement or technique, take it as slowly as you need to. Rushing as you learn doesn't help build technique—it undermines it, because it compromises your Workout and your safety. Speed and flow are the icing on the cake, and they come easily once you've got the proper form.

Work out at the level that's appropriate for you. That means you should be able to:

◻ complete your Workout

◻ maintain a level of intensity that will keep your heart rate within your target heart rate zone (please see page 53 before you begin the Workout)

◻ return to your resting state after about ten minutes of active Cooldown

If you cannot meet those requirements, your current Workout may be too challenging for your present fitness level. You need to go back to a less challenging Workout, or, following the tips throughout this book, modify your Workout.

◻ Be sure you complete the Warm-up and the Cooldown portions of the Workout. Extend either of them if you feel you need to.

◻ Follow a realistic and reasonable Workout schedule. You will probably get the most all-around benefit from working out three times a week or every other day. (See page 27 for more on this.)

Stop your Workout and get medical attention immediately any time you:

◻ feel pain in your chest, arm, jaw, or shoulder

◻ faint, experience lightheadedness, or feel dizzy

◻ experience an unusual or rapid heartbeat

◻ have trouble catching your breath

◻ experience nausea

◻ have unexplained, sudden, or persistent pain, stiffness, or soreness anywhere in your body

◻ have any other symptom that is unusual for you, uncomfortable, or worrisome

With knowledge, patience, practice, awareness, common sense—and a lot of sweat!—you'll be doing Tae-Bo and feeling great now and for years to come. You've got the will. Now you've got *The Tae-Bo Way*. Let's get to work.

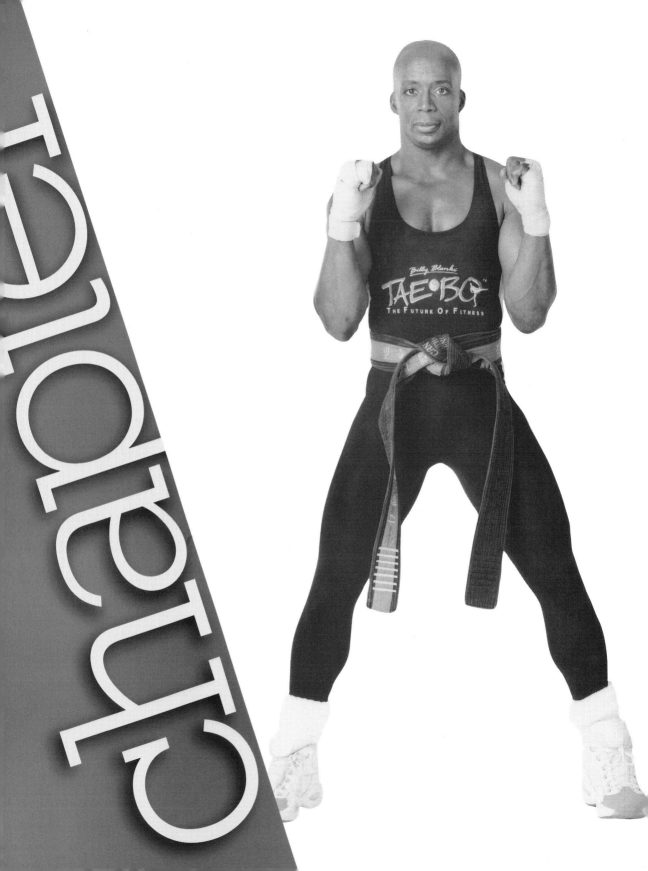

one

The Tae-Bo Way

Are You Ready to Change Your Life?

It doesn't matter who you are, how old you are, what kind of shape you're in, or how much you weigh. It doesn't matter how many other exercise programs you've started and quit. It doesn't even matter that you think you hate exercise. My promise to you is exactly the same. If you give me a chance to show you how powerful you truly are, how committed you can be, how great you can feel, I'll show you the way—**The Tae-Bo Way**.

You may have recently discovered Tae-Bo, but I created it nearly twenty years ago. And I will be teaching it for the rest of my life, because I believe in Tae-Bo—as an exercise program and as a force for personal change. That's why I'm dedicated to bringing Tae-Bo to as many people as possible. The Tae-Bo Workout videotapes were just one way to share the Tae-Bo experience. Now I offer you this book, *The Tae-Bo Way*, the first and only official guide to Tae-Bo.

Here you'll find a step-by-step guide to the Basic Techniques of the Workout, plus the knowledge and insight, and the tips and the tricks that will keep your Workout fresh and make it more fun. I also answer questions I'm often asked about Tae-Bo and explain what you need to know to go beyond the videotapes to make your Tae-Bo Workout your own. Just as important, though, I've written about the philosophy behind Tae-Bo. I'll teach you to tap into and to master those invisible forces inside each of us—will, determination, commitment, and discipline—that can help us win the battle for physical fitness.

This is not a book about "diet and exercise" or a "makeover plan." I'm not going to tell you "how to lose weight" or "how to change your body." I don't believe you can develop "a body for life" without also developing the spirit and the mind to go with it. Don't look here for the names of magic supplements and miracle foods, because I don't believe those things exist.

Instead, I'm going to teach you something even better: how to take control of your Workout and become your own teacher. I wrote this book because it's impossible for me to personally teach each person who wants to learn Tae-Bo. But even if I were standing over your shoulder right now, the teacher would still be you.

What Is Tae-Bo?

Tae-Bo is an exercise program that combines the best of several different disciplines. Tae-Bo brings together the self-awareness and discipline of the martial arts, the rhythm and grace of dance, and the focus and power of boxing. I chose the word "tae," which means "foot and leg" in Korean, because many of the movements emphasize the lower body; "bo" is a shortened form of the word "box." To me, each letter of "Tae-Bo" has significance as well, because they stand for the qualities that Tae-Bo both demands and develops:

T represents *total commitment* to whatever you do

A represents *awareness* of yourself and the world

E represents *excellence,* the truest goal in anything you do

B represents the *body* as a force for total change

O represents *obedience* to your will and your true desire for change

Always remember as you work out: There isn't anything Tae-Bo asks of you that it will not return to you. As it tests your will, it strengthens it. As it pushes your body, it builds it. As it challenges your spirit, it embraces it.

Because Tae-Bo requires strength, endurance, focus, and technique, it engages your mind and your spirit as well as your body. Later, I'll tell you more about how I came to blend them together and how Tae-Bo has evolved since then. But, as you'll see, Tae-Bo is about much more than moving your body and getting in shape.

I know that Tae-Bo will change not only the way you feel and the way you look, but the way you think. I believe that if you give me the chance to show you Tae-Bo, I can show you the way to change your life. And I believed that just as strongly back when I was holding my first classes in 1982 as I do today, when hundreds of thousands of people are doing Tae-Bo. The incredible success of Tae-Bo these past few years has inspired me to reach for even more, to go beyond what I can teach you in a class and through my videotapes. Now it's up to you. Before you begin your journey, let me tell you a little about my own.

Believe in Yourself—Your Whole Self

No one who comes to the Billy Blanks World Karate Center in Sherman Oaks, California, can miss the words written on its walls:

> **Faith without works is dead.**
> **Dead are works without faith.**

Think about what that means. To me, it means that the action that we take based on our faith brings our faith to life. And the faith that we have in what we do gives what we do value and purpose. I believe this is the key to success in every aspect of life.

This is a lesson I've been learning all my life, because I was not always the Billy Blanks you see today. In fact, as a child, I was very aware that most people around me didn't think I'd ever amount to much. I was thirty-seven before I was diagnosed with dyslexia. So through all my school years, I was misunderstood by teachers and placed in special-education classrooms, because they thought I was mentally slow. They didn't understand that where other people saw words that spoke to them, I saw a mess of jumbled-up lines that meant nothing.

Growing up poor, with a limited education, it might seem that I had everything going against me. But I never saw it that way. I was the fourth of fifteen children born to my parents, Isaac and Mabeline Blanks. Even though we didn't have many material things, I never understood how poor we were until I was older. When I think back on my childhood in Erie, Pennsylvania, what I remember most is the love and discipline my parents raised us with. My parents' strength and dedication to each other and to their children set the course for my own life. Not a day goes by that I don't recall my father telling me, "Billy, you have to work hard for everything you want. It's never going to come easy." My father worked in a manufacturing plant and held a second job driving a garbage truck. He taught me that no matter what you did, you did it well.

My family loved and believed in me, but beyond that, I don't think anyone else had any great hopes for me. I was smart enough to know I didn't belong in a special-education classroom, to know that I was capable of learning more. But I didn't understand then that there was a way to teach me. Instead, I wondered if what the teachers said about me was true. I was embarrassed about having to ride the smaller special-education bus to school, while my brothers and friends rode the regular-size school bus.

Sports were important in my hometown, and each of my brothers made his mark as an athlete. But that seemed beyond me too. I was born with tendons that were unusually short and tight, so I had a limited range of motion. There isn't a medical term for this condition, but to give you an example of how much it limited me physically, I could not sit on the floor with my knees bent under me and my rear end resting on my heels. I just couldn't stretch that far. I was so uncoordinated that I literally could not walk and chew gum at the same time.

Not only was I shy and self-conscious, I was awkward too. And it seemed like everyone else I knew had found that one special thing they could excel at, something that gave them confidence and made them feel good about themselves. One day, I found mine.

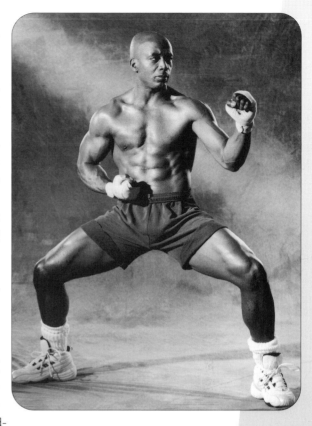

I was about twelve years old when I first saw martial-arts legend Bruce Lee. He played Kato, the Green Hornet's crime-fighting partner in the TV series *The Green Hornet.* The show was silly, but each time Kato took down a villain in a flurry of punches and flying kicks, the true Bruce Lee came through. I was inspired by Lee's determination, speed, and skill. I wanted to be able to do what he did with his body. But more than that, I wanted to feel the same confidence and sense of purpose I saw in him. So I decided I would become a world martial-arts champion. When my mother heard me say that, she said, "Billy, just go sit down."

But I didn't sit down. I found a karate class at a local recreation center and began taking lessons. My karate teacher told me he didn't think I'd last very long, so I guess he let me come back just to humor me. And I kept coming back and working harder than I'd ever worked before. It was soon clear that my physical limitations had to be overcome. But how?

One day, I saw a model of a skeleton and realized that there was no limit to how the bones and joints could be moved and positioned. If all there was to my body was bones, I thought, I could raise my heel to my head. But my muscles and tendons were in the way. I knew that if I could stretch and strengthen those, there was no limit to what my body could do. So I worked on stretching and strengthening my body. Since I couldn't read well, my body became my book and my teacher. I needed to know the names of every muscle and what each one did. I learned everything I could about the mechanics of the body, the purely physical side. I explored how far I could push myself, past discomfort and through pain.

Every day I tried to go farther than I'd gone the day before. Whether I was practicing a stance, a punch, or a kick, even if I'd done it a million times, I was always thinking, always questioning myself. How did that feel? How was it different from the last one? What would happen if I moved my arm a little this way or relaxed my elbow a little that way? I pushed myself as far as I could go, and then farther. I chose to go through "the fire," as I call it, again and again and again. Sure, I had a teacher, but my real inspiration came from inside me. Within a few years of these trials and tribulations, I had physically transformed myself.

It's important to remember that even though the evidence of what I'd done was physical, the transformation went far deeper. I was working for something, and I had faith that I'd achieve it, but I didn't know when or how. It was not my body but my will that pushed me to do better and to be better. The more will I needed to keep going, the stronger my will became. Even so, that young Billy Blanks

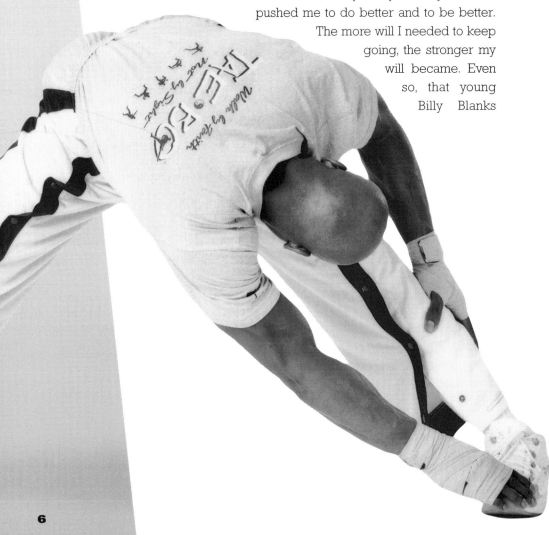

still wasn't a young man you'd pick out of a crowd and say, "He's going to make it." I had a long way to go.

Then one day my life changed forever. My instructor simply said to me, "Billy, you're going to be a black belt today." (In most cases, you must pass tests of skill before you receive a belt. In true martial-arts tradition, however, a teacher considers many aspects of a student's personality and skill and awards belts as he sees fit.) I was sixteen, and from the moment he tied that belt around my waist, everything about me changed. I went from being the kid all the teachers and guidance counselors told "You're going to be a bum," to a young man full of promise and potential. After that, I truly believed there was nothing I couldn't do. I'd learned that in changing my body on the outside, I'd changed Billy the man on the inside. All the confidence I'd lost because of the things I couldn't do as a kid was redeemed now that I had found one thing that I could do. Within a few years, I began competing in local karate tournaments—and winning. Eventually, I would attain a seventh-degree black belt in tae kwon do, as well as black belts in five other forms of martial arts. And, just as I told everyone that I would—and as I'd promised myself—eventually I did become a world karate champion, seven times over.

Calling on the Spirit to Change the Body

In karate I found a new language, a new way to communicate with the world. The stronger I became, and the more confident I became in myself physically, the easier it became for me to talk to people, to express myself, to do those things that everyone for as long as I could remember had been telling me I couldn't do. Now, learning karate didn't teach me how to read well, for example, but it gave me the personal courage and the will to face that challenge later on.

I can break a cement block with my bare hand, but the true source of my strength—and anyone's—lies deeper inside, in the spirit. I knew that if I could touch someone's spirit, I could help that person achieve anything. As painful as my school years were, I learned lessons I still use today. I remember sitting in my special-education classroom and watching my teachers fail to connect with children who were mentally retarded, autistic, and emotionally disturbed. I'd watch these kids, and I could see that each of them had something they wanted to communicate, something they wanted the world to understand about them. No matter what they did with their bodies or their minds, they were still spirits inside. But no one was looking. No one was listening. All my life, I always told myself that if I were ever blessed to be in a position where I could help someone else, I would never turn away. I would learn to understand the whole person. I would never look at someone's body without seeing their spirit too. Years later, when I taught physical fitness to adults facing those same challenges, I saw how physical activity could help them open up and give them a way to communicate they'd never had before.

I was blessed with the realization that the mind, the body, and the spirit work together. Without my spirit, my mind, and my will, I'd never have lasted through my first karate lesson. And without the confidence I've gained through strengthening myself physically, I'd never have developed the will to meet new challenges or have found the spiritual energy I draw on today. My experience—and those of everyone doing Tae-Bo—proves to me that . . .

Physical Fitness Isn't Just About the Physical

Do you believe that? I do, because if getting in shape and keeping your body healthy were only about the physical, we'd all be in shape right now. We'd eat better and exercise more, and the problem would be solved. But it's not that simple, is it? You're smart. You know what you should be doing and how to do it. Yet many of you don't. Even worse, you're confused about why. Why can't I take off ten, twenty, forty, seventy pounds? Why can't I make myself get on the treadmill, in the pool, on the bike, or on the court a few times a week? The problem is that we are more than just our physical bodies. For all their power, the mind can be confused and the will can be weak.

No wonder we listen to the experts who tell us there's a simple physical solution to our problems. When people talk about why a diet or an exercise program failed, they never blame the unrealistic menu plans or the useless exercise gadget they bought. They never question the hype. They don't ask how it would be possible to eat all you want and still lose weight, or get yourself firm and toned just sitting in a chair, swallowing "fat-blocking" pills. They blame themselves. And they seem to know exactly what part of themselves is to blame: their will. "I have no willpower." "I just can't find the will to get to the gym every day." "My will is just too weak."

In the health-and-fitness business, you hear a lot about

willpower. What nobody tells you is that your will doesn't come with the power already installed. Nobody tells you that no matter how weak you think your will is today, you can make it strong—a force for what you *can* do, not an excuse for what you cannot. And you build your will the same way you build your body—by using it, stretching it, pushing it to its limit and then beyond. Everybody tells you how this product or that belief can change you. Nobody really tells you that you already have the power to change yourself without them. You just need to start putting your will to the test. Like I say, If you have the will—and I believe that you do—I have the way.

I'm a student of human nature. I listen to what people say, and I watch what they do. Most of us don't even realize when we say one thing and do the opposite. Many times people will tell me something about themselves and then do something that contradicts that. For instance, someone might say, "Billy, I'm really committed to getting in shape," but then not work out for three weeks because they couldn't find the time. The problem usually isn't not having enough time. It's usually not having the strength to keep a promise you make to yourself.

People who complain that they have no will—or no time, no energy, no discipline, and so on—are often the same people who live up to commitments and do things for other people. I've seen mothers who have the will, the

Tae-Bo changes you from the inside out.

time, the energy, and the commitment to drive their kids to karate class and sit patiently while their kids work out three times a week, every single week, rain or shine. Yet they can't summon the same focus or find even a little time to help themselves. I've seen successful people from all walks of life, people who take charge of any room they enter, come to me full of doubt and ask, "Billy, do you think I can lose weight?" And I've also seen people you'd never imagine doing something as demanding as Tae-Bo—people in their sixties and seventies, people who are chronically ill or who have disabilities, people who struggle every day—come in and shine. How do you explain a sixty-five-year-old grandmother outperforming a professional athlete in class? Or a quiet, unassuming woman having more strength than a corporate CEO twice her size? To find the answer, you have to look below the surface, beyond what your eyes can see.

What Makes Tae-Bo Different?

The difference—and the key to understanding Tae-Bo—lies with the spirit. Through my years training myself and teaching others, I've seen exercise fads come and go. I know how boring and uninspiring a workout can be. But I also know the power of a good workout to get the body moving, the mind working, and the spirit soaring.

I began developing Tae-Bo around 1976, almost by accident, when I started working out in my basement to a copy of the *Rocky* soundtrack my wife, Gayle, had given me. I created a workout for myself that used classic techniques from martial arts and boxing, then added some dance moves just to make it more interesting. Through the martial arts and the boxing, I was developing speed, strength, balance, coordination, and awareness. The dance worked with that, giving the workout an energy and flow that not only improved coordination and body awareness, but also made a great aerobic workout for my heart. That was important, because despite being in what looked like peak physical condition, my aerobic stamina wasn't as strong as I had thought it would be. For the first time in my life, I was getting a true full-body workout.

Soon my wife and our children, Shellie and Billy, Jr., were adding my new workout to the martial arts they were already doing. (Everyone in my family is accomplished in martial arts, and all have taught Tae-Bo. Shellie, who is the other model in these photographs, was a world champion in tae kwon do at age fourteen.) To support myself while I was still training and competing, I taught classes in martial arts and boxing and the new exercise program I later named Tae-Bo. I offered it first in 1982, in Boston. After we moved to California in 1989, I started teaching it in my garage, then in a small studio in the Los Angeles area. In 1997, we moved to the current Billy Blanks World Karate Center, where I still teach. And in 1998, we released our first Tae-Bo Workout video series.

A Word to Women

I designed Tae-Bo for everyone—women, men, and kids. But it's always had a special appeal for women. This is not an accident. I wanted to give women an exercise program that could make them feel stronger and more confident. Because women usually have good lower-body strength, I adopted elements of tae kwon do, a style of karate that emphasizes kicks. To help women improve what is often their weakest area, the upper body, I added some boxing. And then, because I knew women enjoyed dance and music, I studied ballet, so Tae-Bo would have rhythm and flow.

On a personal level, I admit I was also thinking about Gayle and Shellie. I'd trained for decades to fight in a ring. I had the skill, the strength, and the confidence to walk the streets without worry. I never stopped thinking, though, of how little we teach our mothers, wives, sisters, and daughters about how to defend themselves in a world where there's no ring, no rules, and no referee. While Tae-Bo is not a martial art itself, it does teach you how to punch and how to kick. It trains you to respond mentally and physically, quickly and surely. In Tae-Bo, you discover how powerful your body can be and how to use it to defend your-self. I hope you never find yourself in a situation where you have to call on these skills. However, a key to self-awareness is the realization that anything can happen, and I always believe in being prepared for the unexpected. At the very least, practicing Tae-Bo will give you the body confidence, the awareness, and the reflexes to help

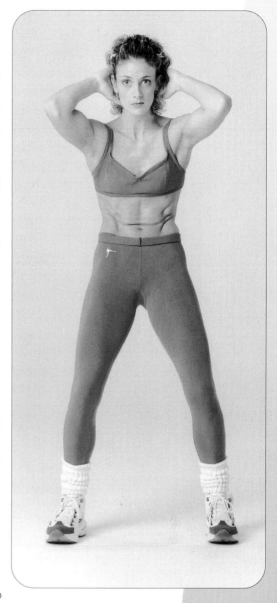

you avoid bad situations. Knowing how to kick and to punch and understanding how to make yourself less vulnerable to attack are the very basics every woman should know.

The Tae-Bo Way: It's About Finding Your Own

If Tae-Bo were simply another exercise program, we could all stop and pat ourselves on the back after we mastered the Advanced Workout. But I know that for myself, for thousands of students I've personally taught across the country, and for the hundreds of thousands who have learned Tae-Bo through the videotapes, Tae-Bo has become much more than just a routine to get in shape. Of course, people do get in shape; some experience dramatic physical changes, losing more than one hundred pounds, for example, or reversing chronic, seemingly incurable health problems. Not a week goes by that I don't hear from a woman who is thrilled with her newfound strength or a man who has the stamina to play sports with his kids for the first time in years. Those are all important aspects of Tae-Bo, but there's even more.

Tae-Bo is also a way of thinking that unites your mind, your heart, and your spirit. Tae-Bo has endured and continues to grow, because no matter what stage you're in—whether you started just yesterday or have been doing it for ten years—I promise you, the Workout will give you challenges and possibilities you never imagined attempting, much less succeeding at. That's why I believe Tae-Bo has no beginning and no end. You can be twenty-one or sixty-one, a champion runner or a world-class couch potato—it doesn't matter where, when, or how you start, as long as you do. (Although if you have a serious or chronic health problem, are overweight, or have not exercised in a while, I recommend that you check with your doctor before you begin any exercise program.) As you'll see in this book, you can sit in a chair and learn how to do a modified Front Kick. Because Tae-Bo teaches you to focus on your technique, it's actually safer than many other exercise programs—especially those that are loosely based on Tae-Bo—that encourage you to blindly "go for it" without teaching you how to move your body safely.

The beauty of the Tae-Bo Workout is that it's your own. You set your goals, you decide how far to push yourself and what you need to achieve to improve your body, your mind, and your spirit. Remember: There is no final destination on this journey, no one goal that marks the end of the road. You can set goals along the way: Maybe in three months, or six months, or a year, you want to have the strength and the stamina to complete the full Advanced Workout videotape without stopping to march. But even after you've achieved that, you can work on other goals inside the Workout. If you can do five sets of eight Side Kicks, don't stop there. You can always improve your technique, or kick higher, or recover more cleanly, or pause the tape and add a sixth set of eight, or create a punch–Side Kick combination for a seventh set.

I've always noticed that most people come into the Billy Blanks World Karate Center to take their first Tae-Bo class with a specific goal. They may come to us to lose weight, get stronger, or get into shape. But within a few Workouts, everyone seems to forget why they came there in the first place. Suddenly it's not about squeezing into those old jeans or lowering their blood pressure. They're there to do the work, to push themselves—physically, mentally, and spiritually—through the fire. And then they discover and grab hold of a lasting goal, one they can believe in forever. The pounds, the waistline, the stress that triggers overeating—they all seem to take care of themselves. That's because students discover the power of Tae-Bo to change them from the inside out.

I've seen the joy and happiness in a student's face the first time he makes it through a whole Workout without skipping any sets. I've seen the surprise when the five-hundredth kick goes higher than you ever dreamed. That sense of accomplishment and strength and the confidence you develop shine through. You can believe me, because I see it happening every day. And I believe it can happen for you too.

No matter how long you work at Tae-Bo, no matter how well you refine your technique or increase your stamina, there will be something new to think about or work toward. And while you may become very good at Tae-Bo, I promise you, there will always be new challenges, if you want them. After all the years I've trained and done Tae-Bo, I still can't get past fifteen or twenty minutes of teaching a class without sweating.

I've always had faith that if each person gave Tae-Bo a chance, they'd discover the same exciting, energizing power I did. I'm still amazed by the dedication and passion students bring to Tae-Bo. From the stage of the Billy Blanks World Karate Center, I see faces I've known for five, ten years. I've seen people change and grow through Tae-Bo. I've witnessed how it's touched people's lives in ways that have nothing to do with exercising. I may not know you, but I know that you have a spirit and that you have will.

It's my hope that through this book I can offer you the knowledge, the insight, and the inspiration to help you keep Tae-Bo part of your life forever. So welcome to Tae-Bo. Thank you for giving me this opportunity to help you learn more about yourself, your Workout, and the Tae-Bo Way.

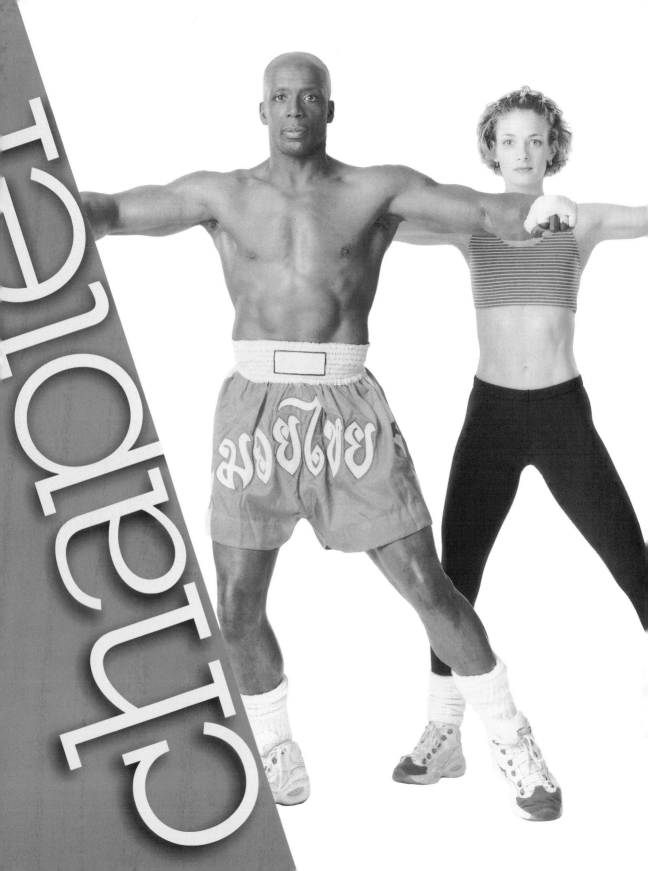

TWO

The Tae-Bo Way
of Thinking

Before you get too distracted by all the moving and sweating you see in Tae-Bo, remember this: You have to use your mind to do Tae-Bo. I designed this Workout deliberately to make it impossible to do correctly without thinking and paying attention. Just as you always have your guard up physically, I want you to always have your guard up mentally too.

One way to improve mental focus is to push yourself to your physical limits. That means working through fatigue, never giving up as long as you can continue working out safely. Always be aware of what you're feeling and learn what it means. Be sensible.

You could get some insight into why Tae-Bo challenges physical limits if you could take a class at the Billy Blanks World Karate Center. You'd find a no-frills exercise floor that's a little warmer, a little muggier, and a little more crowded than you might expect. Sure, we could turn up the air-conditioning or limit the class size. But I don't do that, because I believe that the classes teach students about more than just working out. Tae-Bo isn't about what you can do when your Workout is easy. It's designed to show you what you can do when the going gets tough.

When you do Tae-Bo, you have to think, and you have to stay sharp. And that contradicts what some people think exercise is all about. I've come across people who say one of their favorite things about working out is that it gives them a chance *not* to think. These are people whose workout is nothing more than physical. They may change themselves on the outside, but they're not working anything on the inside.

There's no such thing as "trying," there's only doing.

I know that working out on the physical level alone is not enough. You can be in great shape, but if there's nothing going on between you and your workout, it's never going to last and you'll never feel as good about it as you should. Now, you could do Tae-Bo solely on the physical level and just go through the motions. But I promise you: That would not be Tae-Bo.

You Have the Power to Change

Let's be honest: You can change yourself on the outside. It might take some time, some effort, and maybe some money too, but you can do it. There's a world full of diets, exercise gadgets, and plastic surgeons. But is what's on the outside really the problem? If it were, people either

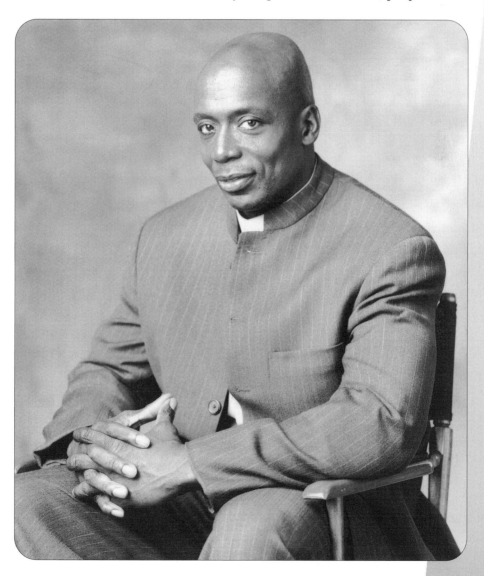

would never get out of shape, or they would lose weight once or take one series of exercise classes, then never think about their bodies again.

Every day I see people who are in great shape on the outside, with "perfect" bodies and beautiful faces. But that's only the outside. Inside, they're torn up by self-doubt, unhappiness, and worry. If the outside change was really all they needed to stay motivated, any physical improvement would be permanent. They'd find what worked for them and stick with it happily. But that's not what happens. No matter how great the results of a new exercise program, one day it ends, and you're

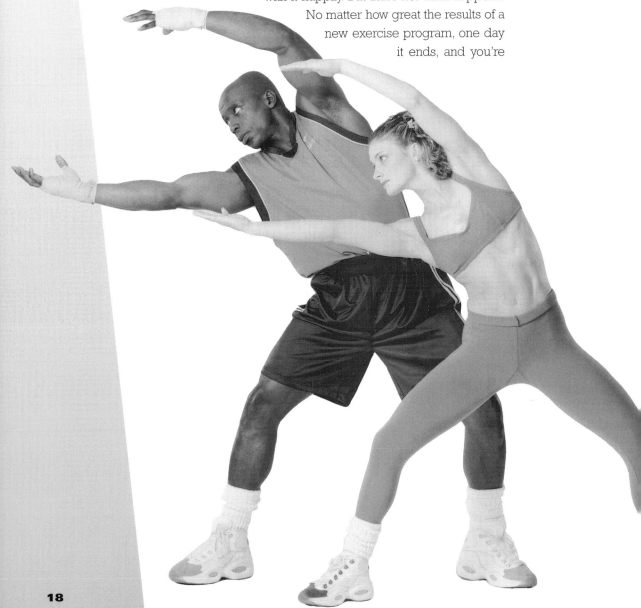

back where you started. Sometimes you're even worse off—more out of shape, more unhappy with yourself—than when you started.

Finding Motivation That Lasts

I believe that most of us try to change ourselves because we need self-assurance. But it's not what we think of ourselves that pushes most of us to exercise and take care of ourselves—it's what we worry that other people think about us. That might be a strong motivation to get started, but it's an emotional one, and emotions usually weaken with time. On the other hand, if you feel good about yourself inside, I truly believe that the outside will take care of itself.

That might sound strange to you. It might sound too easy or too soft, like you might not have to really work for it. With Tae-Bo, believe me, you will be working for it. But you'll be working for the right reasons, toward the right goals.

Part of the problem is how we think about working out. Yes, a good workout is hard and challenging. But are those bad things? Let me ask you this: What would make you feel better about yourself—doing something easy that you've done a hundred times, or achieving something you never thought you could? You know the answer. Everybody wants to improve in their lives. So why do we run away from challenges? I think it's because we fear how much worse we would feel if we failed. But what is failure? To me, it's giving up before you ever begin. It's letting your past rule your future. It's accepting what you don't want. If you were in a restaurant, and the waiter brought you steak when you ordered fish, you wouldn't think twice: You'd send it back. You would get what you wanted and you wouldn't settle for less.

Yet some of you are settling for other things in your life, things that are far more important and have far more serious consequences than what you're eating for dinner. I think people sometimes settle for the boring workout, the lack of results, and the endless dieting because facing a new challenge seems harder. But ask yourself: How easy is it to feel that your body is out of your control? How easy is it to face yourself each day and know that you want something better? And I don't mean what most people would call a perfect body. I mean what you want on the inside: more energy, more strength, more power, more focus, more of a reason to feel good about yourself.

And, as you're achieving all that, there's the bonus: a healthy, great-looking you on the outside too.

I'm not going to lie to you: It's hard to change. It's easy to keep going along, never pushing beyond your limits, never challenging yourself. There are days when I don't feel like getting out of bed and going to my studio. But I do it, because I know I'll be a better and stronger person for it. And it's not because I'll have exercised my body. It's because I'll have exercised my will. And a strong will can overcome anything.

See Your Workout in a Positive Light

Here's a question I ask all my students: What do you think you have to do to get into shape? I usually get these answers: Work hard, be dedicated. Okay, I say. Now, do you think you have to sacrifice to get in shape? Most students immediately say yes. Some might add that working out takes discipline, even punishment. And they truly believe it. Doesn't sound like much fun, does it?

"Why do you think you have to sacrifice to be fit?" I ask. "You should never sacrifice to be fit." This statement always surprises them. Usually a student will reply, "But if you don't sacrifice for your work-out, if you don't punish yourself by spending more time in the gym and less time eating desserts, how will you get in shape?" Like so

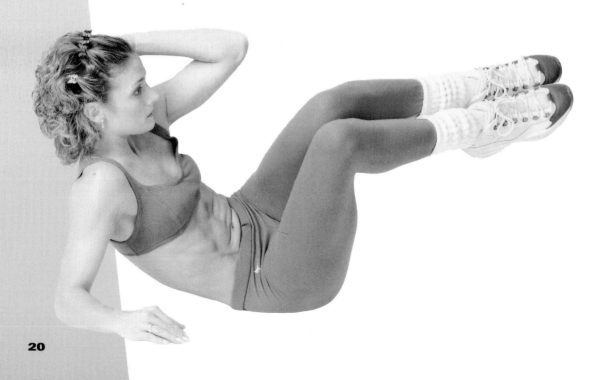

many people, they believe you can't enjoy your workout. Or if you do enjoy it, it can't be hard enough to do any good. Or if the workout is hard, you have to hate it. This kind of negative thinking sets you

Whenever you face a challenge, always ask yourself, "How much better will I be after I succeed?"

up to fail. If you come to any workout—including Tae-Bo—thinking like this, you're finished before you start.

To change your body, you first need to change your mind about exercise and see your workout in a positive light. I've noticed fitness trainers "give up" on their clients, thinking that they are weak, lazy, or not committed. After those fitness trainers showed their clients what to do, they thought their job was done. If you got on the bike, picked up the weights, or stuck with the class, great. If you didn't, there was always another customer coming through the door.

I saw it differently. I saw that the failure wasn't in the student but in a negative approach to fitness, because physical fitness is not really about the physical. It's about a whole person. It's about you. So forget everything you've ever learned about what it takes to get in shape. You know that negative thinking doesn't work, because if it did, we'd all be in shape right now. Besides, do you really believe that you can feel good about something that makes you feel bad? Of course you don't. And once you start sacrificing—your time, your energy, your pleasure—to get in shape, it's only human nature to look for a reward. That's where sacrifice turns to sabotage. That's why diets crash in uncontrolled splurges (followed by self-defeating guilt) and exercise programs end with that one missed class that snowballs into twenty (followed by more self-defeating guilt). Or you can mix and match it: You deserve that hot fudge sundae because your exercise class was so boring. Or you didn't eat the hot fudge sundae, so you can skip the class.

It's a no-win situation all the way around, because the natural response to sacrificing for something is to resent it. And as you might know from your own experience, each time we fail makes it that much harder to believe we can succeed the next time.

Don't set yourself up to fail. Before you make your first move, change your thinking. Set yourself up to conquer—your body, your thoughts, your will.

It's About Your Spirit

We live in a world where too many people have lost sight of what they really are and how blessed we each are to have the power to change. Instead we focus on how we look, how smart we are, how much we earn, and so on, even though these things can be easily lost in an instant. Our bodies are as fragile as butterfly wings. In the end, when the physical body dies, we're each left with the essence of who we are—of who we always were and always will be: a spirit. How can any fitness idea or program that deals with only the physical body succeed? It can't.

What do we mean when we say, "I believe"? You can believe on many different levels. One way to believe is to know that something is true. I believe that working out will improve my health. I know that it's true. I believe it. But I'm not doing anything about it. Or we say we have faith in something, which is another way of saying that we believe that something exists or that something will happen. Yet we don't act on that, either. You might have faith that if you worked out every day for two weeks, you'd feel a lot better than you do right now. But you're still not working out.

Remember those words on my wall: Faith without works is dead. Knowledge, faith, and belief are dead unless you act on them. And how you act on them is just as important. It all begins with your attitude. Did you know you can change the tone of your voice just by smiling? Try it. Say something without smiling, and then say it again with a smile on your face.

I'm a great believer in the power of words and the power of names. Faith comes by hearing. If you say something out loud, you're more likely to believe it, and if you believe it, you're more likely to act on it. I believe that we are motivated by the words that we speak and the words that we hear.

It's not always easy to feel positive, but going through your days in a constant state of "whatever" only keeps you from appreciating life and respecting yourself. These days, some people think that kind of thinking is cool, but it's not. Slowly but surely, it will influence and sabotage everything you do, and you will become careless and unaware in everything. I feel so strongly about a positive attitude that if I see someone at the front of the class who's working out half-heartedly or carelessly, I ask them to move to the back. Or even leave.

When I say, "Be a conqueror," I mean be a person who makes things happen, not a person things just seem to happen to. Find your power, and use it to better yourself and to help others.

I've watched people start exercise programs, then quit. The problem wasn't that they had given up on fitness. It was that they were giving up on themselves. So when you come to work out, show yourself the respect and consideration you deserve. Before you turn that critical eye on your reflection in the mirror, give yourself a smile. Tell yourself what a great job you're going to do instead of complaining to yourself about how hard it will be or how many workouts you skipped last week. Remember: You're working too hard not to feel good about the person you're working for—yourself.

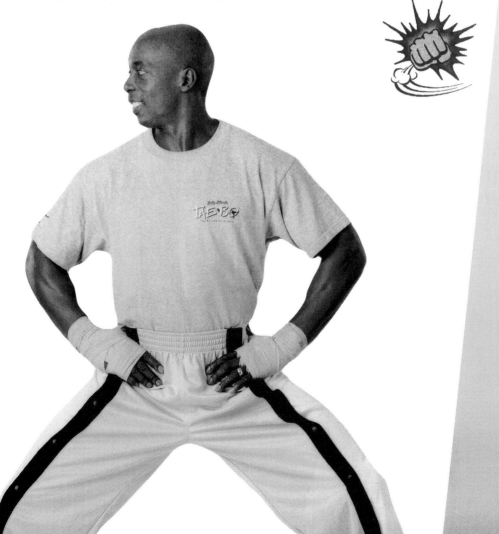

23

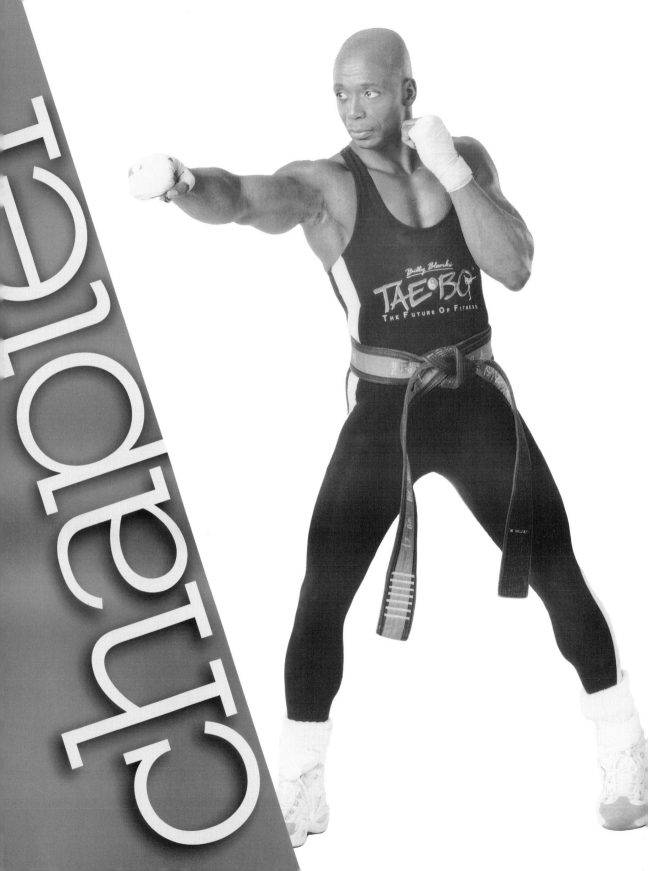

three

The Tae-Bo Workout:
Getting Started

Tae-Bo is different from any other workout, and it's a difference I guarantee you will feel the first time you try it. To do the Tae-Bo Workout correctly and to get the most out of it, you have to exercise a part of you that doesn't get much attention on the gym floor. That's your mind. No matter how strong you are, no matter how fit you are, if you aren't concentrating on your technique, you aren't really doing Tae-Bo.

Tae-Bo demands that you develop a keen sense of self-awareness. That means you must concentrate on what every part of your body is doing. Everything you do in Tae-Bo involves your whole body. You'll learn that the key to executing the perfect kick depends on more than just how you move your leg. Where you look with your eyes, where you stand, how you hold your arms, and how well you control your abdominal muscles—all these things and many more determine the quality of your kick.

Many beginning students of Tae-Bo find this full-body focus their biggest challenge. This is especially true if you haven't worked out much before. You might be surprised to learn that this can be a problem for people who come to Tae-Bo in good condition too. That's because most other fitness programs either focus on one area of the body at a time, or they use exercises (for example, step classes) or equipment (such as treadmills) that encourage you to mentally zone out. I designed Tae-Bo so it won't let you zone out. Is it harder? Sure. But it's worth it. You will feel and see the difference in your body *and* in your attitude.

You'll probably find that it takes a while to learn how to hold that mental focus *and* work out. That's okay. Speed and agility are important in Tae-Bo, but you will achieve them with time and practice. To master Tae-Bo, you have to master technique. And technique always comes first. If you have to work a little bit slower, that's fine. If you can kick only as high as your knee when you start, that's fine too. Keep working on executing every movement consciously, deliberately, and correctly. Think positively. Don't focus on what you're not able to do today. Instead, focus on how that slower warm-up or that lower kick is preparing you to progress tomorrow.

Frequently Asked Questions

Will Tae-Bo work for me?

I won't even answer that question, because the real question is this: Will I work for Tae-Bo? If you've got the will, I've got the way. I can't tell you if you have the will today or how hard you'll work to develop it tomorrow. Only you know that. If you're serious about it, though, Tae-Bo will work with you, and you will achieve your goals.

Do you have to be strong, flexible, or coordinated to do Tae-Bo?

Tae-Bo doesn't ask anything of you that it doesn't give you in return. Beginning Tae-Bo with these strengths may make the Workout easier for you than it would be for someone without them. However, as I've said before, being in good shape now doesn't necessarily guarantee that you'll breeze through Tae-Bo. And not being in good shape doesn't mean that you can't do Tae-Bo. We each have such a wide range of abilities and skills. You might be thirty pounds overweight with amazing balance. Or you might be a highly trained athlete who stumbles through the combinations at first. You might come to Tae-Bo with good muscle tone and strength but little flexibility. Or you might have great energy but a weak sense of rhythm. Or you might have a great sense of rhythm but little awareness of what your body is doing. That's the beauty and the challenge of being human.

The important thing to remember about Tae-Bo is that you don't need to bring anything to your Workout but determination, discipline, and a willingness to listen, watch, learn, and work toward change. Unlike some other exercise programs, Tae-Bo doesn't demand flexibility, control, coordination, strength, and endurance—it helps you build them. That's why you should never give up on any move, combination, or Workout without giving it your best shot. The moment when you feel you can't hold a position for one more second is the moment you are gaining balance. That last set of reps that you think you'll never get through is the set that's building your endurance. Doing what you can't do is what makes it something that you can do.

How often should I do Tae-Bo?

You can get the full benefit of the Tae-Bo Workout by doing it three times a week. Especially when you start out, your body will need a day between Workouts to recover. On those off days, you might want to do some stretching if your muscles feel a little tight or you have a mild, general soreness.

Some people love to jump right into it. I'm happy when people tell me that they love Tae-Bo so much they do it every day. However, you don't need to do it every day. For one thing, when it comes to working out, more often doesn't always translate into greater benefits. Working out six times a week will not improve your overall fitness level twice as quickly as working out three times a week.

That's because working out improves your fitness several different ways. Understanding how Tae-Bo works will help you plan the Workout schedule that's best for you, one that will help you reach your personal fitness goals.

Basically, Tae-Bo is effective in three areas:

1 The intense aerobic activity burns calories and can reduce stored fat. That's how you lose weight or maintain a good body weight.

2 The aerobic activity also provides a good workout for your heart, making it stronger and more efficient.

3 The controlled movement and whole-body focus tone and strengthen your muscles. That's also how you lose weight and reshape your muscles.

Every time you work out, you burn calories, and after a certain point, you begin to break down and use stored fat for energy. If you think only in terms of how many calories and how much fat you're burning, the more you do the Workout, the quicker you'll see those results. You should know, however, that working out more often doesn't necessarily tone, firm, or build muscle more quickly. That's because building muscle is a longer, ongoing process that occurs mostly when your body is at rest. Exercising jump-starts the process, but your muscles need some down time for it to be completed. So in terms of strengthening your muscles, you may see more benefits by working out three or four times a week than you would by working out every single day. Remember, though, that over the course of a week, you would burn more calories with daily Workouts.

You also need to be honest with yourself. You know your strengths and your limitations. You know your history. Think about how you've approached working out before. Did you take it slow and steady? Did you find a schedule that was reasonable, so you had time to work out without feeling that you were taking time away from something else? Or did you jump in, full of enthusiasm and unrealistic goals, only to quit after a few weeks or months because your workout was taking too much time and effort? Or did you injure yourself? I have to be honest: I'm always a little concerned about anyone who announces, "I've been doing the tapes twice a day for the past three weeks!" I know from experience that few people can continue at that pace for long. And when they give up—because it takes too much time, or they get bored, or they strain a muscle—they give up all the way. The improvements they've made will fade over the next few months; then what will they have gained?

It's better to be realistic about working out. Start off doing Tae-Bo two or three times a week. If you want to do more than that, great. But just be sure you're doing it for the right reasons and that you're not setting yourself up to burn out. Enthusiasm is great. Just remember what I said about being motivated by emotion: There will come a day when the emotion fades and you'll need a stronger, steadier force to motivate you. You'll need your will.

You may be working out too much if:

- you start making excuses to skip your Workout
- you skip a whole week of working out daily instead of trying to work out three or four days each week
- you find yourself going on automatic pilot during the Workout and making mistakes
- you don't feel that you are making any improvements in terms of technique or endurance

What are other exercises and activities I can do in addition to Tae-Bo?

I believe that anything you do to improve and strengthen your body is good. That's why I never tell my students that one type of exercise is better than another. I might warn you that something I'm about to teach may be different from what you've learned from another form of exercise, but that's only because it can be a safety issue. For example, you never want to lunge and let your knee cover your toe in Tae-Bo, even though this is an acceptable and safe move in dance. (You'll see more of these reminders later when we get to the actual movements in "The Basic Techniques.")

Physical fitness is not just about the physical.

The one other workout I'd recommend to enhance Tae-Bo is weight training. That's because in weight training, you focus on working specific muscle groups. Also, anything you do to strengthen your body will help you in Tae-Bo. Some women avoid weight training because they worry that it will make them bulk up. You don't need to worry about that, because, for men, the classic bodybuilder physique comes as much from the male hormone testosterone as it does from the act of pumping iron. (The women bodybuilders you see with "masculine" forms have been working out for years at an extreme level.) Working out with weights a few times a week will firm, tone, and strengthen your muscles without adding bulk.

When you're doing weight training, remember that how you work is as important as what you work. Doing fewer reps with heavier weights will build muscle bulk and strength. On the other hand, doing more reps with lighter weights will give you strength and tone without making your muscles that much larger. This is good to know, especially if you want to work on problem areas that you don't want to make bigger, like the upper thighs or the butt.

Not surprisingly, many people who start doing Tae-Bo often study martial arts too. I encourage anyone with an interest in martial arts to pursue it with the best instructor you can find. If you do study martial arts, or have in the past, you should be aware that even though most of Tae-Bo is based on martial-arts movements and techniques, some have been modified and are not strictly the same.

How long after I start doing Tae-Bo can I expect to see results?

You are unique, and your experience with Tae-Bo is too. Because almost anyone can do Tae-Bo and because the Workout can change you in so many different ways, it's impossible to set a timetable for specific improvements. How quickly you lose weight and inches, or how easily you tone and firm your muscles, will depend on other things you do as well. How often you do the Workout, the level of intensity you reach, and which Workout you're doing will all influence how much weight you lose. Obviously, what you eat, how much rest you get, and other health and lifestyle factors also play a role. I can tell you, though, that doing Tae-Bo even two or three times a week will make a difference in how you feel and how you look.

Lost weight and inches are easy to see. Some other important benefits of Tae-Bo cannot be seen with the eyes but are just as real. Endurance, strength, heightened awareness, confidence, agility, and balance all improve with Tae-Bo. After a few Workouts, don't be surprised to find yourself standing a little taller, walking with more confidence, and just feeling better about yourself all around. Nobody's come up with a way to measure and chart things like keener awareness. Nobody's figured out how increasing your fitness makes housework a little less tiring and that long commute not quite so hard on your back. Yet these are all the invisible benefits reported to me by thousands of people who do Tae-Bo.

Am I going to sweat?

You'd better! If you've been telling your friends, "I'm doing Tae-Bo and not even breaking a sweat," you have one of two possible problems. Either the Workout you're doing is not challenging enough for you and you should move on to the next level, or you're not really doing Tae-Bo the Tae-Bo Way.

As a student and as a teacher, I've always believed that one of the most dispiriting, discouraging things a teacher can do is compare his students to himself. I think that breaks people's spirits and discourages them, so I don't do that. But you'll notice that if I'm sweating twenty minutes into teaching a class, everyone should be sweating. If you're not working up a sweat after twenty minutes, you need to seriously think about what you're doing. Are you doing all the movements? Are you striving for intensity? Are you working your entire body? Are you following the right technique and working toward proper form? Are you moving using the full range of motion? Are you fully controlling your every move? Are you in balance? Does your Workout have rhythm and flow? Are you pushing yourself to and beyond your limitations? If you're doing all this, you've got to be sweating!

Another thing: Being able to do the Workout too easily is not a goal of Tae-Bo. Long before a particular Workout gets to be that easy for you, you should be challenging yourself with something far more demanding. That's the Tae-Bo Way.

What should I wear when I'm doing Tae-Bo?

You should wear whatever feels comfortable, keeps you warm (or cool, depending on what you prefer), and won't get in your way. You want to be sure that whatever you're wearing allows you to move freely and have a full range of motion. You should be sweating, so you will want to avoid fabrics that don't breathe. Some people like cotton, because it's absorbent and cool. Others prefer the newer synthetics that breathe and draw moisture away from the skin and keep you feeling dry.

Whether you wear shoes or not is up to you. Some people prefer to work out barefoot because it makes their legs lighter for kicks, they can pivot more freely, and they have better balance because they can feel the floor. My daughter, Shellie, for example, often works out without shoes. I always wear shoes, because I'm more comfortable having some support in my arches and ankles. The extra cushioning you get in a good pair of shoes helps those who have knee or foot problems.

If you wear shoes, choose a style that's lightweight and supports your ankles without coming up too high. Before you buy a pair, try a few kicks and pivots to see how easily they allow you to move on the floor. Check the soles and the treads. If you'll be working out on a carpeted surface, look for a smoother sole, since deep treads can catch on carpeting and cause you to stress your ankles, knees, and hips.

Finally, a note for women: There's a lot of movement in Tae-Bo, so I recommend that women with larger bustlines wear a good sports bra. The type that flattens and supports is usually best. Look for a sports bra that's either totally or partially made from a stretchy synthetic like Lycra or Spandex. Bras that are 100 percent cotton are softer, but they don't provide much support. For those who are larger-busted, a constructed cup-style bra especially designed for sports is a good choice. I've found that it often improves the Workout too, because jiggling makes some women feel self-conscious, and they restrict their movement to avoid it.

Tae-Bo isn't about how much better you can feel or how much better you can look. It's about how much better you can be.

Are there any special requirements for the room where I'll be doing Tae-Bo?

All you need is enough room to work out without hitting something. You might be surprised to learn how little space that can be. As long as you can move four long strides in every direction, you'll be fine. Keep the room at a comfortable temperature and have plenty of fresh air. Have enough water, or whatever you're drinking, available and your VCR remote close at hand, so you can stop the tape if you need to.

One thing to consider is the type of floor you work out on. Many newer homes and apartments have floors laid over cement, and these can be hard on your feet and knees. Try working out on a well-padded carpet or while wearing shoes with good support. Some people like working out on a bare floor, and a wooden floor can be the most comfortable surface of all. Just remember that bare wood, tile, or linoleum is slippery when wet. Don't be surprised if you sweat enough to create a few barely noticeable but hazardous damp patches around you. Keep a towel handy and pause now and then to wipe the floor dry.

Is it okay to drink something while I'm working out?

Yes, it is. And not only during your Workout—before and after too. Your body needs a consistent supply of water to replace what you lose throughout the day. We tend to think that we lose most of our water through sweating or through urination. But you're also losing water when you breathe. Very few people drink nearly as much water as they should each day, even when they're not working out. For good health, you should be drinking at least eight to ten eight-ounce glasses of water every day. If you're drinking only when you feel thirsty, you're dehydrating your body. By the time thirst kicks in, you're already behind one or two glasses. Even minor dehydration can cause muscle cramps, overheating, dizziness, and excessive fatigue. To give you an idea of how important water is, remember that your body could survive weeks without food, but only a few days without water.

I always recommend that people drink water instead of other beverages, but, again, it's your decision. Some people like the extra energy boost they get from the sugars in sports drinks and juices. Others feel the need to replace minerals lost through sweating with sports drinks that contain sodium and electrolytes. Yet some people find that drinking anything other than water while they're actively working out slows them down or gives them stomach cramps. Whatever you drink, be sure to avoid beverages that contain caffeine (because your heart will be beating fast enough anyway) or are carbonated (because carbonation can produce uncomfortable stomach gas).

What should I eat before I do Tae-Bo?

My basic advice for what to eat when you're doing Tae-Bo is this: Eat a light, complex-carbohydrate snack about an hour *before* you work out, and eat protein *after* you work out. That's because complex-carbohydrate foods provide your body with a slow, steady stream of energy for your Workout. Afterward, high-protein foods provide the building blocks to repair and renew your muscles. You should also avoid fats, because they are hard to digest and can slow you down. And foods high in sugar (candy, sweets, soda, and so on) will provide a quick energy rush, but they may cause your blood sugar to drop just as quickly, leaving you with even less energy than you had before. *Never work out hungry.*

Now, beyond that, everyone is different. Although many people find that eating protein slows them down before a Workout, there are some who tire more easily if they don't. I believe you should listen to your body and do what you feel is right for you. You might be shocked to learn that my favorite post-Workout snack is red licorice!

Complex-Carbohydrate Snacks

Carbohydrates are divided into simple carbohydrates and complex carbohydrates. Simple carbohydrates include sugar in all its forms and almost anything that has a high sugar content, such as sweetened breakfast cereals, cake, cookies, candy, fruit drinks, and so on. Simple-carbohydrate foods give a quick energy boost because your body digests them easily and dumps sugar into the bloodstream in one big batch, but

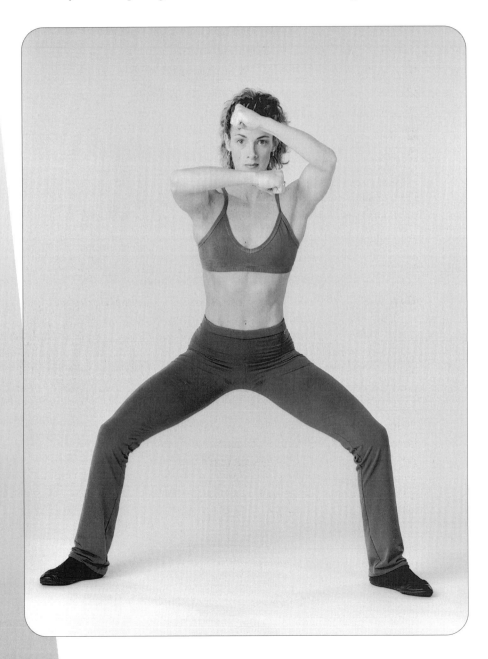

the downside is that the blood sugar peak you hit with these foods doesn't last very long, and once your blood sugar drops again, you may feel like you have even less energy than you did before.

Complex carbohydrates affect your body differently. They take longer to digest, so your body releases sugar into the blood in a slow, steady stream over a longer period. Eating complex-carbohydrate snacks about an hour before you work out will help you keep your energy up without a sudden drop in blood sugar and that tired feeling that comes with it. Complex carbohydrates are usually low in fat and contain fiber.

Some good complex-carbohydrate snacks include:

- unsweetened or very lightly sweetened breakfast cereal
- whole-wheat or whole-grain bread or pasta
- rice, rice cakes
- nuts
- seeds
- fruit
- vegetables
- beans
- potatoes
- pizza

How many calories will I burn doing the Tae-Bo Workout?

If you're of average weight for your height, in reasonably good shape, and work out hard enough to really sweat and get your heart rate up for at least twenty minutes, you're probably burning anywhere from 300 to more than 600 calories an hour. One fitness expert estimated that certain people could burn up to 800 calories during an hour of Tae-Bo.

How many calories you burn depends on a number of different factors: your weight, the length and intensity of your Workout, the percentage of your body weight that's muscle as opposed to fat, your general level of fitness, and your basic metabolism. Each person's body is unique, but most people find that the combination of aerobic exercise and strength training (in the floor work and repetitions) could burn both the calories they eat today and the fat they've stored. We have received hundreds of letters from people who have dropped from 10 to 110 pounds doing Tae-Bo without changing their diet.

One great benefit of doing Tae-Bo and getting in shape is that muscle burns more calories than fat tissue, even when you're sitting down doing nothing. The higher the ratio of muscle to fat, the better your metabolism works, and the more calories you burn just going through your day.

What about dieting while I'm doing Tae-Bo?

I'm all for healthy eating, but everyone seems to have a different opinion about what makes a healthy diet. I believe that as long as you're working out and burning the calories, there's no reason to restrict what you eat. Of course, everything should be done in moderation. Most people who are doing Tae-Bo regularly find that they feel so good about themselves it gets easier and easier to skip the chips, sweets, sodas, and fried foods. And they do it without feeling deprived or like they're making a sacrifice. When you deprive yourself and start resenting the positive changes you're making, you're sowing the seeds for sabotage. I'd rather see someone eat that piece of chocolate cake, fully enjoy it, and then work it off than think of it as something to fear, obsess over, and then feel guilty about. And I truly believe that if you spent as much time working out as you may be spending reading food labels, shopping for wonder-drug supplements, or rearranging your lifestyle to conform to the latest diet, you'd be much more pleased with the results.

You can follow a moderate diet program—one geared to help you lose no more than one to two pounds a week—and do Tae-Bo. Crash diets, high-protein diets, and starvation diets (fewer than 1,000 calories a day) do not provide the energy your body needs to maintain good health and still have the 300 to 600 calories the Tae-Bo Workout will burn. You have to work out at a certain level of intensity before your body starts metabolizing stored fat. The moment you begin working out, your body burns the calories that are quickly available from the carbohydrates and sugars in your blood. Throughout the Workout, however, your body needs the instant energy that comes only from what you have eaten that day.

When calories are burned, they produce energy. When they don't get burned, they get stored as fat. Every excess pound of body fat represents about 3,500 extra, unused calories. Where does it come from? After you've eaten all the calories your body needs to function each day, all it takes is the caloric equivalent of:

- ◘ thirty-five tablespoons of butter, or
- ◘ ten super-rich Häagen-Dazs chocolate-covered chocolate ice cream pops, or
- ◘ eight large orders of fast-food french fries, or
- ◘ thirty-five eight-ounce glasses of regular cola, or
- ◘ six and a half Big Macs

to gain a pound.

Most people don't overeat only one type of food, so this illustration is unrealistic. Usually the problem is eating more calories—50 here, 100 there—than we burn each day. But I think you can see how the calories can pile up before you know it.

Whether you're eating too much fat or no fat, whether you're living on junk food or the purest organic food you can find, whether you're a vegetarian or a steak-and-potatoes person, whether you're eating for your body type, food combining, following a commercial diet plan, or making it up as you go along—it doesn't matter.

A calorie is a calorie, and your body processes each calorie exactly the same way. Your body takes carbohydrates (which includes sugars) and fats and burns them for your immediate energy needs.

Change the way you think and you can change your life.

Whatever is left over is stored as body fat and takes the form of extra inches and pounds. Protein is used first to build and repair your body tissues (including muscle), and is sometimes used for energy, if carbohydrates and fats are not available. Some people believe that protein calories cannot be stored as body fat, but that's not true. If you eat more calories than you need in protein, those calories also will turn to fat. Your only choice, then, about how to handle those extra calories boils down to this: Burn them through exercise, or wear them.

I hesitate to focus too much on food, because some people would like to think that if they just ate less, they wouldn't need to exercise. This kind of thinking can lead to unhealthy, even dangerous eating habits. We're seeing too many people—even little girls and boys—who have taken concerns about weight and diet to unhealthy, even deadly extremes. If you're a parent, you should be aware of the messages you send your children every time you say "I shouldn't be eating this," "I'm so fat," or "I have no self-control anyway, so pass me the chips."

I'm all for healthy eating habits, but the truth is, the secret to health isn't so much what you put in your body as what you do with your body. Eating too few calories may actually make it harder for you to lose weight, because your body will hold on to whatever body fat you do have to protect itself from starving. (Only your mind knows that you're choosing to skip meals or eat fewer calories than your body needs to function well. As far as your body's concerned, that calorie shortage may never end.)

As with anything, please use common sense. You may not be eating enough calories if: you're feeling faint or extremely fatigued early in the Workout and/or for hours afterward; you're working out but the pounds aren't budging; you're not seeing the improvements in strength and muscle tone after a few weeks. Check your diet.

Why is it more important to exercise than to diet?

Diet and exercise are two distinct parts of a healthy lifestyle that we mix together in our minds and then constantly try to balance: "If I work out today, I can have that fudge sundae," or "I'm only letting myself have diet sodas and three diet shakes today, so I'll skip the Workout." Neither approach is effective nor healthy. It's best if you can have a reasonably healthy diet and a solid exercise program. But too many people make the mistake of using one—often diet—to make up for not doing the other. I've seen too many people who would almost literally starve their bodies if it meant they could avoid breaking a sweat.

Extreme dieting is never a good substitute for exercise. No one who's following a starvation diet (fewer than 1,000 calories a day) has the energy to maintain their basic body functions and follow a challenging exercise program. The fact is, you need calories to produce the energy you need to work out vigorously enough to burn stored fat. Got that? I feel so strongly about this that if I see a student who looks undernourished or too thin, I will pull him aside and talk to him. If I can't convince him to eat reasonably, I won't allow him to return to my studio until he does. It's a matter of safety.

Dieting is never the whole answer to any problem. It may help you control your weight, but nothing you put in your mouth can maintain, build, tone, or strengthen your muscles, or improve your balance and endurance. Eating a healthy, low-fat diet can keep you from developing some forms of heart disease, but it cannot make your heart stronger. Your body is much more than a calorie-processing vehicle that carries your head around. It was designed to move. When you deprive yourself in what you eat and then deny your body the joy and the power of movement, your spirit suffers too. Never forget: It's all about more than just the physical.

But there's even more good news. Researchers have found that people who try to lose weight by dieting alone without exercising are more likely to gain it back once the diet ends. People who exercise, however, find it easier to lose the weight and keep it off. Another reason to exercise is that moving your body feels good, while dieting usually does not. That's why it's much easier to make exercise a part of your life than to make dieting a way of life. Most of us could

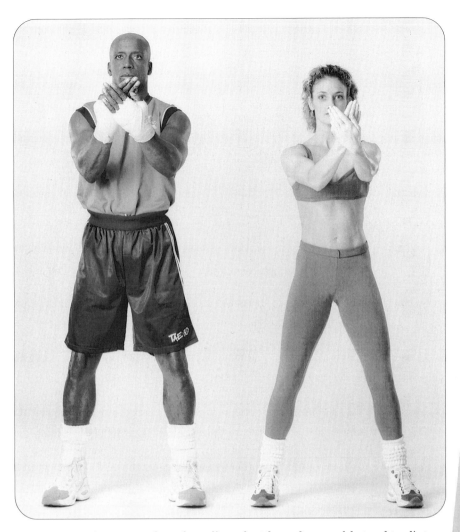

exercise every day of our lives, but few of us could stand to diet for more than a few weeks.

How Tae-Bo Works: Using the Videotapes

The original Tae-Bo video library consists of four videotapes:

Instructional Workout

Basic Workout

Advanced Workout

The Eight-Minute Workout

These were designed to be used in that order, and you should not move up to the next tape in the series until you have mastered the information and the techniques in the tapes that came before it. Now, I know there are some who take one look at the Basic or the Advanced Workout and let their eyes do

*If you've got
the will, I've got
the way.*

their thinking for them. After all, you might reason, it looks easy enough. Tae-Bo may look easy. It's not.

Even if you already work out, even if you've studied martial arts, you must take the time to learn what I teach in the Instructional tape. It contains techniques and tips that everyone needs to work out intelligently. As you learn more about Tae-Bo and see how the movements are broken down and explained in the chapters that follow, you'll see that every part of any movement is important. Grace, speed, and endurance often depend on how well you execute the small details of your moves. You'll learn how the angle of your right foot can make or break a left Side Kick, and how looking in the wrong direction can mess up a punch.

If you injure yourself while working out, it may be because you are not always using good technique. You may be rushing, failing to start and finish your moves from the right position, or forgetting the little things, such as pointing your toe when you kick or glancing over your shoulder before a Back Kick. Always remember: In Tae-Bo, it's safety first. Know your own fitness level and be aware of your limitations. Work slowly at your own pace, and don't move forward with more repetitions or a more challenging Workout until you are ready. That means you have to always be aware and know what your body is doing. Be careful about getting so deeply into it that you lose control. Anytime you start to feel yourself shift into cruise control, hit the brakes and back up.

In Tae-Bo class, I test my students' control by shouting "Stop!" without warning. Just like in the game freeze tag, wherever they are when I say stop, they freeze. If they can't keep their balance, then they were not moving with control. If you can hold your body perfectly still—even if you were in the middle of a kick or a punch—you're doing Tae-Bo. You might test yourself by having someone signal you to stop at random during your Workout, or trying to hold your position for about ten seconds before you answer the door or the phone if you're interrupted. Another thing you could do is set an egg timer or the alarm on your watch without looking, so you don't know when it will go off, and freeze when you hear it.

When am I ready to move from the Instructional videotape to the Basic Workout?

No one knows you better than you do, so ultimately this is your decision. Whatever you do, please don't let your enthusiasm get the best of you. The purpose of the Instructional tape is to help you build a foundation. If you don't take the time today to learn everything on it, you won't be getting the most out of Tae-Bo in the future. I know many people are anxious to move to the first full Workout, but keep these points in mind:

- You can use the Instructional tape as a Workout by alternating sides, even though the demonstration uses only one. After you've watched the tape a few times, you'll be able to switch sides easily. You can work on a new move during those times when I'm explaining a technique that may not apply to you (such as using a chair for balance).

- Don't be self-conscious or embarrassed to stop the tape, rewind, and try something again, as many times as you have to.

- One way to gauge what you've learned is to watch the tape without the sound and try to identify each move. If you can tell a Hook from a Cross, a Roundhouse Kick from a Side Kick visually, you're on the right track.

- Another way to measure your progress is to stop the tape toward the end of each exercise and do two, three, four, or five additional sets of eight. Or you might try double-timing half the sets.

- See where you fall in your target heart rate zone (see chart in Chapter 4). If your endurance has improved to the point that this Workout isn't raising your heart rate up to at least 70 percent of your maximum heart rate (MHR), it isn't challenging enough for you from a cardiovascular perspective. (For more information on target heart rate and maximum heart rate, see page 52.)

- If you can fully execute each technique and movement without ever once looking at the television screen during the tape, you're ready to move on.

Now, I often hear people who have not worked out much recently complain that the Instructional tape is too easy for them, that they didn't even break a sweat or raise their heart rate. This might be true of someone who is studying martial arts or who trains vigorously in some other exercise. But to be honest with you, most beginners who think they're flying through that tape are more likely flailing their arms and their legs, instead of punching and really kicking with full control. I know from watching the Beginner classes we teach that it takes time for most people to learn how to execute the moves with the full body, in complete balance and in perfect time. If you can't do that with this tape, you'll be struggling through the next.

If you think you're ready to move up, test yourself. Watch the Basic Workout several times and take the time to just listen and watch. Then stop your Instructional tape before the Cooldown, try to do the first ten or fifteen minutes of the Basic Workout, then go back to the Instructional Cooldown. If you're comfortable with that, add a few more minutes over a week or so until you're confident you can do the whole Basic Workout safely from start to finish. You're on your way.

When am I ready to move from the Basic Workout to the Advanced Workout?

Basically, once you've mastered the techniques, you feel that your fitness level has improved, and you feel you're ready for a greater challenge, consider moving up. Ask yourself the same questions you asked before moving up from the Instructional tape. Check how you're doing in terms of your cardiovascular fitness by comparing your target heart rate from when you first started doing Tae-Bo to your current one. Having a moderately low heart rate while you're working out—say between 50 and 60 percent of your maximum heart rate—means one of two things: Either you're not working out as intensely as you think you are, or you have become so fit and your heart is so efficient that you're not being challenged. You might want to stick to the Basic Workout a little while longer, but add sets or do more of your sets in double time, or concentrate more on working your whole body until you bring your heart rate closer to 75 percent of your full capacity.

Stop your Basic tape before the Cooldown and pop in the Advanced Workout for ten or fifteen minutes. Check your heart rate. If you're working out at a higher rate and still breathing correctly (hard and fast but not gasping for breath), you're ready for the next step.

You can always go back too.

We each have our strengths and weaknesses. It's possible that you might be ready to move up to the next tape and still have a few rough spots to work out. Put on some music and practice the kick, the punch, or the combination that you can't quite master yet. And I always urge everyone—even people who have been doing Tae-Bo for five, ten years—to go back to the Instructional tape every month or so. Believe me, the more you learn about Tae-Bo, the more you'll be able to learn. Experience gives you a greater understanding of what makes a Hook not a Cross and what gives footwork definition, energy, and flow. I learn something new every single day.

How can I tell if I'm ready for the Eight-Minute Workout?

If you're comfortable with the Advanced Workout, try it. If you've been doing Tae-Bo for a while and still find it a little too challenging, that's okay. It was designed to be a tough Workout, and many people prefer the longer Workouts. The purpose of the Eight-Minute Workout is to give people pressed for time a good, total-body Workout that makes it easy to stay on track with their fitness goals. It's intended to be used with the other Tae-Bo Workouts, and it's not—as some people think—the ultimate test of your Tae-Bo skills or their endurance. If you never do the Eight-Minute Workout, you haven't lost anything in terms of skill. However, I encourage everyone to try it at least once every now and then to measure their progress. You might be surprised to find how well you do.

I find it difficult to stay motivated on my own. But no one is offering real Tae-Bo classes where I live. Any suggestions?

I wish everyone could have the opportunity to experience Tae-Bo in a big room with at least a few dozen other students. There's an energy, an electricity in a class that even I can't stay away from. That's why you'll still find me teaching classes several times a day. I could have allowed Tae-Bo to be taught everywhere by anyone who felt like hanging up a sign. But I've chosen instead to limit the number of Tae-Bo instructors I personally train and certify. I want to ensure that everyone who takes a Tae-Bo class learns to do it correctly and safely. To date, there are fewer than thirty certified Tae-Bo instructors teaching true Tae-Bo classes around the United States. We're working on a certification program that will increase the number of certified Tae-Bo instructors. It takes time, because every certified instructor is someone whose training I have overseen personally, and I promise that it will always be that way.

If you're having a hard time staying motivated, I suggest getting a Workout buddy or two. Many people find this helps them stay motivated in any exercise program. It works especially well with Tae-Bo, because you can cheer each other on and be a second pair of eyes for your buddy when it comes to technique. That's not to say you'll be teaching each other, but it can be easier to remember all the different parts of any move if somebody else is there to yell out "Get your guard up" or "Turn your heel." If you are someone's Workout buddy, remember to help them the Tae-Bo Way: Inspire and suggest, but don't criticize.

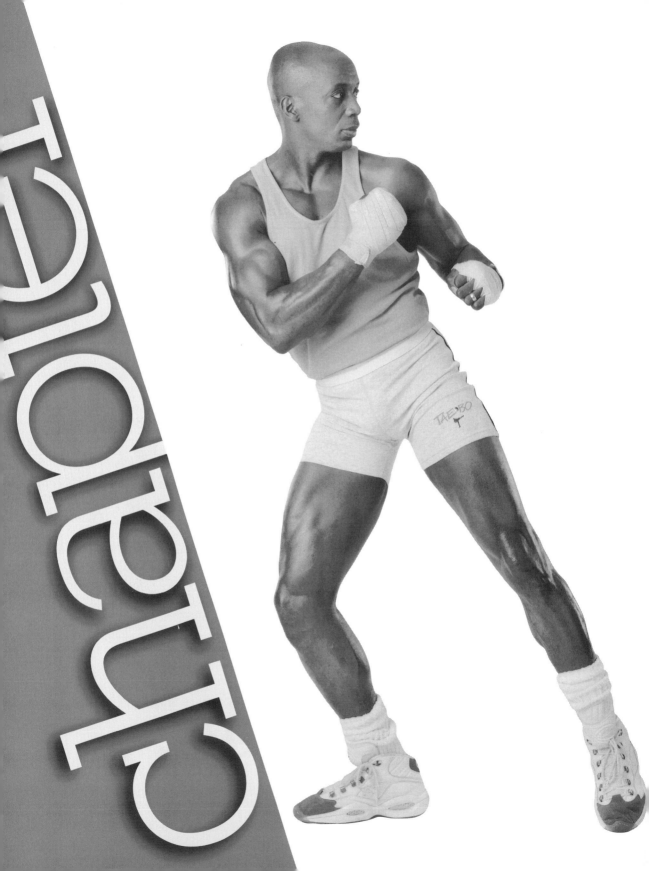

The Tae-Bo Way of Fitness:
Know Your Body

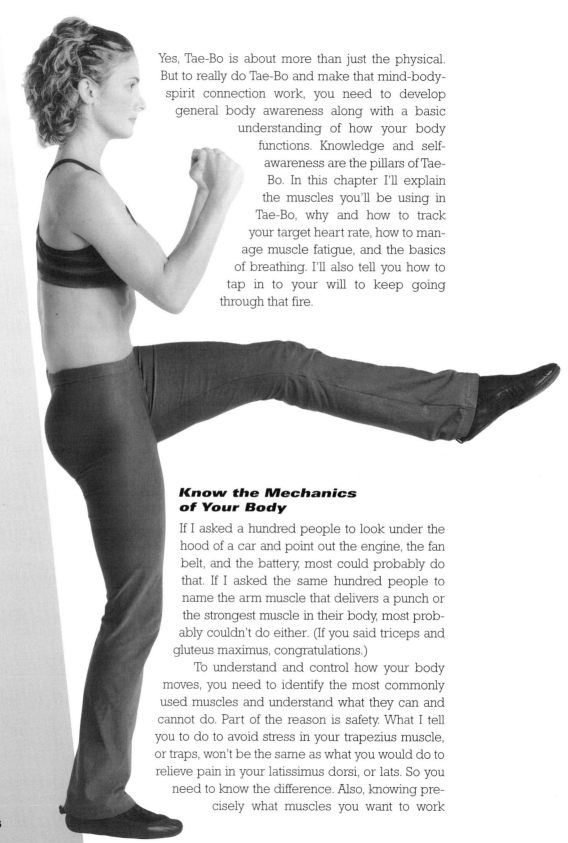

Yes, Tae-Bo is about more than just the physical. But to really do Tae-Bo and make that mind-body-spirit connection work, you need to develop general body awareness along with a basic understanding of how your body functions. Knowledge and self-awareness are the pillars of Tae-Bo. In this chapter I'll explain the muscles you'll be using in Tae-Bo, why and how to track your target heart rate, how to manage muscle fatigue, and the basics of breathing. I'll also tell you how to tap in to your will to keep going through that fire.

Know the Mechanics of Your Body

If I asked a hundred people to look under the hood of a car and point out the engine, the fan belt, and the battery, most could probably do that. If I asked the same hundred people to name the arm muscle that delivers a punch or the strongest muscle in their body, most probably couldn't do either. (If you said triceps and gluteus maximus, congratulations.)

To understand and control how your body moves, you need to identify the most commonly used muscles and understand what they can and cannot do. Part of the reason is safety. What I tell you to do to avoid stress in your trapezius muscle, or traps, won't be the same as what you would do to relieve pain in your latissimus dorsi, or lats. So you need to know the difference. Also, knowing precisely what muscles you want to work makes your Workout more efficient and more effective. A good example is ab work (and I know how much you all love ab work!). When we say "abs," we're really referring to several different sets of muscles. Most ab exercises target one group over the others. If you don't know which ones you're supposed to be working, you won't get the best results for the effort you're making.

Good technique starts in your mind. That's why I'm always reminding you to maintain your focus. Begin and complete one move in one thought before going on to the next move and the next thought. People get confused and start messing up when they move *between* thoughts. In other words, if you're just beginning to deliver a Side Kick, but your mind races ahead to touching down that foot before you've even recovered your leg, your foot is going to drop to the floor like a rock. It won't look good, and it won't feel good either. So you need a clear, sharp focus to guide your body.

A teacher is only a guide. A good student becomes his own teacher.

How can you have clear thoughts about how to move your body when you don't know the names of the muscles you're working? Now, you might wonder, *Well, I'm moving my arm. What else do I need to know?* To do Tae-Bo, you need to know a lot more, because I'm not asking you to just "move your arm." I'm asking you to concentrate and focus on moving a particular part of your arm when you deliver a punch, and then to focus on moving a different part of your arm when you recover the motion. Now, I'm not saying you have to get a degree in anatomy. You only need to know about a dozen major muscles or muscle groups, so when I say "Work those lats," or "Tighten those glutes," we're all speaking the same language.

Tae-Bo also teaches you about the strengths and the limitations of these areas. You are spirit, and your body is a temple, but it's also the most awesome machine. Even after all the years I've been training, I'm still amazed by what the human body can do. Exploring your body's potential takes responsibility and knowledge too. It doesn't matter what kind of injury you have or what you were doing when you got it. Most sports- and exercise-related injuries begin with ignorance and lack of awareness. Every part of your body has limitations. Knees are great for bending, but they're not designed to move laterally, from side to side. That's why you have to pivot. Hips are incredible ball-and-socket joints, and you can use that to your advantage

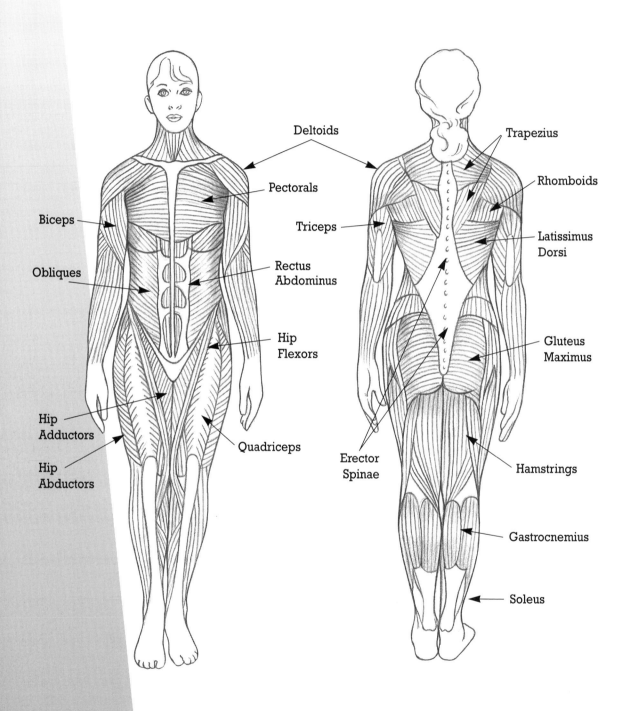

Deltoids

Pectorals

Biceps

Triceps

Obliques

Rectus
Abdominus

Hip
Flexors

Hip
Adductors

Hip
Abductors

Quadriceps

Trapezius

Rhomboids

Latissimus
Dorsi

Gluteus
Maximus

Erector
Spinae

Hamstrings

Gastrocnemius

Soleus

when you turn your hip up before a Roundhouse Kick. If, on the other hand, you think of your hip as a hinge that swings straight up to your side, your technique and your body will both suffer.

Tae-Bo is effective because it works so many different muscles with each move. Here are the muscles and the muscle groups I talk about in the Workout. It helps if you learn to identify these muscles and think of them as pushing muscles or pulling muscles. Later, you'll learn how you can use your breathing to work with your movements by inhaling when you pull and exhaling when you push.

The Abdominals

Whatever move you're doing in Tae-Bo, you should always be working and tightening your abs. We all know that tight, toned abs look great, but they're much more important than that. Your abdominal muscles stabilize and support your entire body. That stability gives you that solid foundation that makes it easier to control all of your movements. A good example of this is the role your abdominals play in good kicking technique. Another thing good abs can do for you is make those full-body moves and pivots go smoothly.

Except to think about how much better we'd like our abs to look, most people don't give them too much thought. One reason Tae-Bo is so effective is that you have to be thinking about your abs just about all the time. I tell my students to think of their torso as a pillar that everything else they do radiates from. When I can, I demonstrate what I mean by standing against a pillar while punching or kicking. You can see my arms and legs move, but the rest of my body, from my head to my hips, is upright, steady, and controlled. (Of course, there are some moves that call for a different position; we'll talk about those later in the book.) You need strong abs not only to help you deliver a punch or a kick, but also to recover the motion and to pivot fully.

The two types of abdominal muscles you'll hear me talking about most are the rectus abdominus and the obliques. The rectus abdominus, the big, flat muscle that covers the front of your abdomen from your lower ribs to your pubic bone, allows you to bend forward, remain upright, and keep your balance. The obliques are the muscles at your sides that help you bend, pivot, and twist.

Correct breathing with abdominal work is simple. Anytime you contract your abdominal muscles or bend forward or to the side, you should exhale.

The Arm and Shoulder Muscles

There are more than twenty different muscles in your arm, but you need to know about three: biceps (at the front top of your extended upper arm), triceps (at the back and bottom of your extended upper arm), and the deltoids (in your upper arm and shoulder). Your biceps is the muscle that pops up when you "make a muscle." Your biceps causes your elbow to bend, so that also makes it the muscle you'll be using to keep your elbow slightly bent and stop your arm short of full extension when you punch. This is a pulling muscle.

The triceps is a pushing muscle. Women often want to develop good triceps because poor muscle tone in that area is the cause of flabby upper arms. Anytime you extend your arm, pound something with your fist, do a pushup, or push something away from you, like a door or a stroller, the triceps is at work. In Tae-Bo, the triceps is the muscle that delivers a punch.

The deltoids, or delts, are important because they're the muscles that allow you to move your arm up, down, forward, and back, and rotate it, as we do in the Warm-up. If you're not controlling your punches, you may feel strain in this area.

The Chest

The main muscles of your chest are the pectorals (pectoralis major and pectoralis minor), or "pecs" for short. Both are pushing muscles. The pectoralis major is the chest muscle that delivers your punch (large, triangle-shaped muscles in your upper back—your latissimus dorsi, or lats—pull the punch back and recover it). The pectoralis minor brings your shoulder forward and downward. Pushups are great for building these muscles, especially if you lower your body to the ground slowly.

The Back

When most people think of back pain, they think of their spine. Most back pain, however, comes from back muscles that are weak or strained. Done properly, Tae-Bo is safe for your back, and it will strengthen and stretch the muscles that cause most of the problems. Anytime you're feeling discomfort in your back, chances are you're not controlling your punches (upper back and neck) or kicks (lower back). Another source of back pain could be failing to pivot fully.

The upper-back muscles I refer to are the trapezius, or traps, one of two large triangle-shaped muscles that stretch from your lower neck to the middle of your back. Your traps help hold your upper body erect and help you lift your arms. When you feel pain in your traps while punching, it's a sign you're either holding up your arms by hunching your shoulders or you're raising your elbows too high.

The rhomboids are smaller muscles that lie along the spine

and reach across to your inner shoulder blade. When you pull your shoulders back, the rhomboids are working for you.

The third group of back muscles is the latissimus dorsi; we just call them lats. Your lats form another large triangle across your back, from just under your armpit and along most of your spine, ending below your waist. Tae-Bo works your lats every time you recover a punch, move your arm up or back, or stand up straight. If you have trouble keeping your shoulders straight and level, your lats need work.

In the lower back, we're most concerned with the erector spinae, or erector, muscles. These run roughly parallel to the spine from top to bottom and are the main supports of the lower back. There's hardly anything you do—stand, sit, walk—that doesn't depend on the erector muscles. You will want to use these muscles correctly and be careful not to strain them through poor technique in your kicks or failing to pivot correctly.

The Hips and Legs

When students reach that point in the Workout where they need their will to pull them through the fire, chances are they're doing legwork. Some people find the ab work the most difficult part of the Workout, but the legwork is often the most challenging because the muscles you're working are so large that they force a lot of blood to flow into them. By understanding which leg muscles Tae-Bo works most, you can learn to work them in ways that will help you stick with the Workout, even when you feel you can't go on.

When you think about kicking, you probably think first about your legs. As you'll see later in the book, the real source of power behind your kicks is having good technique and complete control over your abs, your hips, and your glutes (the gluteus maximus, and the less important gluteus medius and gluteus minimus). The glutes are easy to find; it's your butt. Not only is the gluteus maximus the biggest muscle you have, it's also the strongest. And that's why working it gets you sweating and your heart pumping faster than any other exercise.

Each part of your leg contains several muscles, but the ones we talk about most in Tae-Bo are the hamstrings, the quadriceps (or quads), the abductors, and the adductors. An individual muscle can work alone or with others to move part of your leg. Understanding where these muscles are and what they do will help you isolate them and concentrate on them for the best results. You need these muscles to be strong so you can deliver a strong kick, control it, and recover it smoothly.

Your hamstrings are actually three muscles that run up the back of your leg from the knee to the hip. Strong hamstrings take the pressure off your knees and help prevent injury. They also control how your knee bends, so they're key to kicking correctly. They check your kick and keep your knee from fully extending at the point of impact.

On the front, inner, and outer side of each thigh are the quadriceps, or quads, four powerful muscles that allow you to run, walk, jump, kick, jog, even stand. One links your knee to your pelvis; the other three run from the knee area up along the thighbone. Like hamstrings, quads can protect your knees. One inner-thigh muscle you should be familiar with is the teardrop muscle, the vastus medialis, a quadriceps muscle on the inside of your thigh that helps extend your leg.

In Tae-Bo we don't talk much specifically about the inner-thigh muscles—the adductors—and the outer-thigh muscles—the abductors. But it's easy to remember what they do if you know that the *ab* in abductor means "to draw away from" and the *ad* in adductor means "to pull toward." So abductors help lift and move your leg in directions away from your body, while adductors help your leg move back toward your body. It's easy to understand how important these muscles are to kicking and most of our Floor Work.

Anything you do with your foot is being controlled in part by your calves, those two large muscles that run from your heel up the back of your lower leg to your knee. Your upper-calf muscle is your gastrocnemius; the lower one is your soleus. Every time you flex or point your toes—the smallest but sometimes the most important part of a kick—you're working your calves.

You'll also notice that we often mention the hip flexors. Flexors are muscles that flex joints. Hip flexors are crucial to Tae-Bo, because these are the muscles that raise the leg in Knee Raises and in kicks.

Your Heart and the Target Heart Rate Zone

It's easy to measure the lost weight and inches or the ability to handle a greater number of reps that result from doing Tae-Bo. But other changes are not so easy to measure. You really can't tell how much more you're sweating or how much harder your muscles might be working compared to your last Workout. You can always measure your heart rate, though, to see how you're doing aerobically.

Measuring your heart rate is simple, and something I encourage everyone to learn how to do. In the sixty seconds it takes to check your heart rate, you'll get information that will tell you how well your heart is working and how much stronger you are aerobically. You can also use your heart rate to get an idea of how hard you're working out and then judge if you're ready to push yourself further or if you need to slow up a little. You can get a rough idea of how hard you're working out by

AGE	50% MHR	60% MHR	70% MHR	75% MHR	80% MHR	85% MHR	90% MHR	100% MHR
			HEART RATE, BEATS PER MINUTE					
			TARGET HEART RATE					
15	103	123	144	154	164	174	185	205
16	102	122	143	153	163	173	184	204
17	102	122	142	152	162	173	183	203
18	101	121	141	152	162	172	182	202
19	101	121	141	151	161	171	181	201
20	100	120	140	150	160	170	180	200
21	100	119	139	149	159	169	179	199
22	99	119	139	149	158	168	178	198
23	99	118	138	148	158	167	177	197
24	98	118	137	147	157	167	176	196
25	98	117	137	146	156	166	176	195
26	97	116	136	146	155	165	175	194
27	97	116	135	145	154	164	174	193
28	96	115	134	144	154	163	173	192
29	96	115	134	143	153	162	172	191
30	95	114	133	143	152	162	171	190
31	95	113	132	142	151	161	170	189
32	94	113	132	141	150	160	169	188
33	94	112	131	140	150	159	168	187
34	93	112	130	140	149	158	167	186
35	93	111	130	139	148	157	167	185
36	92	110	129	138	147	156	166	184
37	92	110	128	137	146	156	165	183
38	91	109	127	137	146	155	164	182
39	91	109	127	136	145	154	163	181
40	90	108	126	135	144	153	162	180

CONTINUED...

AGE	50% MHR	60% MHR	70% MHR	75% MHR	80% MHR	85% MHR	90% MHR	100% MHR
			HEART RATE, BEATS PER MINUTE					
			TARGET HEART RATE					
41	90	107	125	134	143	152	161	179
42	89	107	125	134	142	151	160	178
43	89	106	124	133	142	150	159	177
44	88	106	123	132	141	150	158	176
45	88	105	123	131	140	149	158	175
46	87	104	122	131	139	148	157	174
47	87	104	121	130	138	147	156	173
48	86	103	120	129	138	146	155	172
49	86	103	120	128	137	145	154	171
50	85	102	119	128	136	145	153	170
51	85	101	118	127	135	144	152	169
52	84	101	118	126	134	143	151	168
53	84	100	117	125	134	142	150	167
54	83	100	116	125	133	141	149	166
55	83	99	116	124	132	140	149	165
56	82	98	115	123	131	139	148	164
57	82	98	114	122	130	139	147	163
58	81	97	113	122	130	138	146	162
59	81	97	113	121	129	137	145	161
60	80	96	112	120	128	136	144	160
61	80	95	111	119	127	135	143	159
62	79	95	111	119	126	134	142	158
63	79	94	110	118	126	133	141	157
64	78	94	109	117	125	133	140	156

whether you can talk while you're exercising. If you cannot carry on a conversation while you're working out, or you cannot catch your breath without stopping your Workout, you're pushing yourself too hard and should slow down.

You can do exercises that will tone, firm, and build your muscles without increasing your heart rate too much. If you want to burn a lot of calories and strengthen your heart, however, you have to work up to and maintain your pulse within a range known as your target heart rate zone. (You may also see the term "training heart rate zone.") When your heart is beating at 60 to 85 percent of your maximum heart rate, you're in your target heart rate zone and working hard enough to get the full cardiovascular benefit of your Workout. However, it is recommended that you maintain a target heart rate of 75 percent of your maximum heart rate. As your level of fitness improves, you will be able to do the same Workout at a lower heart rate. But when that happens, you need to increase the intensity of your Workout to keep your target heart rate at 75 percent of your maximum heart rate.

Here's how to find your own target heart rate zone:

1 Find your maximum heart rate. One way to do this is to subtract your age from 220. For example, if you're thirty years old, your maximum heart rate would be 190.[1] *Your maximum heart rate is not where you want to be working. The maximum heart rate is the pulse rate where your heart will be working too hard. Never exceed 85 percent of maximum heart rate!*

2 Next, take your maximum heart rate and, using the chart, find the number of beats per minute that fall between 60 and 75 percent of your maximum heart rate. If you're thirty years old, your target heart rate zone would be between 114 (60 percent of your maximum heart rate) and 143 (75 percent of your maximum heart rate).

3 Setting the heart rate you want to work toward depends on what kind of shape you're in, aerobically speaking, when you start Tae-Bo. *You have to remember that you can be fit on the outside—good muscle tone, perfect weight, and*

---

[1] *This method applies only to people whose resting pulse rate is an average of 60 to 70 beats per minute and those who are not taking medication to treat blood-pressure disorders (for example, beta blockers). If you are in extremely good cardiovascular shape, your resting pulse could be as low as in the 40s (because your heart is stronger and is able to move more blood with fewer beats). If you take any medication regularly, it might affect your resting pulse rate, particularly medication for high blood pressure. Talk to your doctor before you begin an exercise program and follow the target heart rate limits he or she recommends.*

great flexibility—and still have a heart in not much better shape than your average couch potato's. In fact, I've seen professional athletes huffing and puffing during Workouts that middle-aged housewives who'd been doing Tae-Bo for a few months breezed through. No matter what shape you look like you're in, unless you've been doing aerobic exercise and working out your heart too, don't assume that you should be working at the upper range of your target heart rate zone to start.

4 You really need to track your heart rate only once or twice each Workout. After you become more familiar with how your body feels at different times, you may know about where you are without taking your pulse. When you start out, though, you need to get to know your heart. Take your pulse (either at your wrist or your jugular in your neck) for ten seconds, then multiply that number by six. Now you know how many times your heart is beating per minute.

5 Until you become more familiar with your heart rate, try writing down your heart rate at a couple of points during each Workout for the first two weeks or so. The more you work out, the higher the heart rate you should be able to work at. You might be struggling at 60 percent today, but soon you'll be on your way to 65, 70, even 75 percent of your maximum heart rate.

Be *SMART* **about your** *HEART*

Working out can be safe for everyone if you take responsibility for yourself. According to the American Heart Association and other authorities, you should talk to your doctor before starting any exercise program or sport if:

- you have been diagnosed with a heart condition or any other chronic illness or condition
- you experience pain or pressure anywhere in your upper body or arms during or right after any physical exercise
- you have experienced chest pain in the last month
- you lose consciousness or fall because of dizziness or lightheadedness
- you have a hard time catching your breath after mild physical activity
- you are now taking or your doctor has recommended that you begin taking medication for high blood pressure or a heart condition
- you have bone or joint problems
- you have not been physically active, lead a sedentary lifestyle, have not worked out in the last three to six months, or are middle-aged or older
- you are pregnant

6 Remember, though, the goal is not to simply get your heart beating faster. You're working to find a perfect balance between the intensity of your Workout and your level of conditioning. If your current level of fitness makes it difficult for you to complete your Workout at 75 percent of your maximum heart rate, you should scale back to 70 percent or lower, or switch to a less challenging Workout.

7 Always take it slow. You're responsible for your Workout, so do the Workout a couple of times and then take your pulse at a few different points. Start by working toward the 60 percent figure and keeping your heart beating at that rate for at least twenty minutes. If you can do that with ease, try to work toward 65, 70, or 75 percent.

8 Always follow the health and safety guidelines in the "Be Smart About Your Heart" box on page 56.

Your target heart rate zone can also be a good indicator of when you're ready to move up to a more challenging Workout. You may not find your Workout aerobically challenging enough for you if:

◘ you've been doing any one of the videotapes and working your entire body but still not raising your heart rate above the 65 percent MHR

◘ you've hit a plateau at 70 percent of your MHR or lower

◘ you can complete the same Workout without increasing your heart rate to 75 percent of your MHR

Here's what you can do: Add more reps to your Workout and/or work out at a higher level of intensity to keep your heart rate around 75 percent of your maximum rate.

On the other hand, tracking your target heart rate can give you one indication that your current Workout is beyond your present aerobic fitness level. You may not be ready for the Workout you've chosen if:

◘ you find yourself tiring very quickly or unable to follow it comfortably

◘ you cannot get through the Workout without slowing down or stopping frequently

◘ you have to quit before the Workout is complete

◘ your heart rate is rising above your target heart rate level, or exceeding 75 percent of your MHR

In this case, you must go back to a less challenging Workout. Remember: Tae-Bo isn't about being able to do the most demanding Workout. The real goal is to do your Workout at a level of intensity that challenges and strengthens you cardiovascularly and also tones, firms, and builds your muscles. But to get the most out of your Tae-Bo Workout, you need to be able to complete it. Working out at an intensity and a target heart rate that's beyond your fitness level and then quitting halfway through or not being able to execute the moves correctly does nothing to improve your fitness and can be dangerous.

Breathing

Students often ask me if there is any special way to breathe while doing Tae-Bo. Now, you've probably tried the Workout or watched a videotape, so you know that you are going to sweat. You may also think that means you should be breathing hard too. Yes, you will be breathing hard, but not in the way you might think. Throughout this book, you'll read a lot about the idea that your body reacts to reaction. That applies to many aspects of Tae-Bo, but here's how it works with breathing.

Take a nice, slow, deep breath, then let it out slowly. How does that make you feel? Probably a little calmer and more relaxed. Part of that is because you're concentrating on the breath more than you might

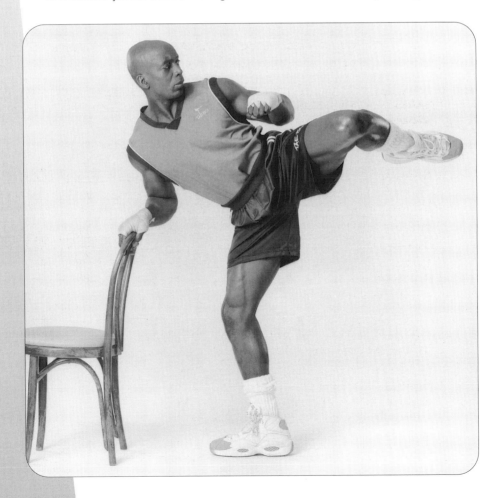

otherwise. But it's also because your ears are hearing and your mind is concentrating on the sound of your breathing. The

same principle applies to your breathing while doing Tae-Bo. If you hear your breathing and it's rhythmic, steady, and quick, that's how you're going to respond. If, on the other hand, you're exaggerating your breaths—breathing deeply, gasping loudly when you inhale, and so on—you're going to respond to that instead and find yourself slowing down, falling out of time, and losing your focus. Breathing like that also signals your body to tighten up, even panic a bit. That's not what you want.

If you're breathing properly throughout the Workout and you're doing the Workout that's right for you, you shouldn't find yourself so short of breath that you need to pause for more than a minute or so. What often happens is that you may be tensing up when you're punching, kicking, or holding a position. Without realizing it, you may not be taking complete breaths, or you may not be breathing at all. Anytime you find yourself taking a big breath after a move, it means you were probably holding your breath a little right before.

You say, "Your body reacts to reaction."
What exactly does that mean? And what
does it have to do with my Workout?

I believe we each have more control over every aspect of ourselves than we can imagine. You can even change the strength of your technique by the words you hear yourself saying. I saw a great example of this when I was teaching a class recently. As we were working on the Roundhouse Kick, some students were having trouble repositioning their feet and legs for the next kick because as they were coming back down into the Horse Stance, they let too much of their weight shift back to the kicking leg. This meant that in that split second before the next kick, they had to quickly redistribute that weight, and this was causing them to lose their balance and fall out of time. For the first few sets, I said "Step, kick, back, down." On "back," the students were placing the kicking foot down on the floor, and on "down," they were stepping to the side with the supporting leg and assuming the Horse Stance. Everyone was trying their hardest, but the technique was still coming up short.

For the next sets, I changed a single word. Instead of saying "back" when the kicking leg came down, I said, "touch." Without giving any more direction, everyone instinctively started touching the kicking foot down lightly between kicks instead of really standing on it with their weight. This kept the weight focused on the supporting leg and kept the kicking leg lighter, so it was coiled and ready for the next kick. The difference in the next sets of Roundhouse Kicks amazed everyone.

Now, part of this had to do with the words we used. But it also had to do with the physical movement of the body. Touching the foot down lightly sends your mind and your body a message that says, "Get ready to go. We're not stopping now!" When that foot drops down heavily and the weight moves to that leg, you'll have a harder time convincing your body that it's not time to rest.

Remember: Anytime you touch your foot lightly or tap it sharply on the floor, take a clear, directed step, pivot fully, focus your eyes and your mind on exactly where you intend to punch or kick, or make a full, complete recovery from a move, you're sending your mind and your body signals. You're telling them to be aware and ready for the next move.

This is why counting out loud is so important. People who know how to count in time can also substitute key words to direct their bodies. One student found she got a better flow in her two-count Back Kick if she told herself "kick, rock it / kick, rock it" instead of "one, two." Others who have trouble getting the hang of alternating punches might want to substitute "left" and "right" for the numbers. Or you can mix them up. A four-punch combination might work better for you if you say "left, left, right, left" instead of "one, two, three, four." Also, don't hesitate to tell yourself other things. You can be saying "Jab, Jab, Jab, Cross" or "one, two, three, four" but also thinking "turn" after the Cross, or "step" as you're Jabbing. Again, it takes time and practice to pull all the elements together, but you can do it.

Throughout the book, and especially in the Basic Techniques chapter, you'll see many tips for making sure that each move you make prepares your body for the next one. When you reach the point where every act sets up a positive reaction, you'll be getting as much energy out of each move as you're expending, and you'll hit that state of flow that some of my students call "addictive" (but in a good way). You'll be doing Tae-Bo on a whole other level.

How to Tell When It's Really Too Hard

I think the question here really should be: How Can I Stop Myself from Quitting Too Soon? I'm a great believer in your power to go beyond your limitations. Most of us are capable of doing more than we think we can. That's why I designed Tae-Bo to really push you to that point where it takes your will to keep your body going. It's a challenge. I'll never tell you that it's not. But it's one you can overcome if you learn to work through your fatigue instead of trying to avoid it. Nobody wants to feel tired, worn out, and stretched to the limit, but, remember, this is just a Workout. Whatever fatigue or stress you feel when you start pushing your body is temporary. Your mind knows you'll feel better after the Workout and that you'll be proud of yourself when you're done. In that moment of weakness, the question isn't whether or not to quit. You aren't going to quit. The question you should be asking yourself is how you're going to tap in to your will to overrule your body, which just can't wait for you to sit down and stop. Remember: You know you're not going to quit. What you need to know is what you've got to do to keep going through the fire.

Do you remember those cartoons where Bugs Bunny is thinking about whether to do the right thing or the wrong thing? On one shoulder, a devil shouts in your ear, telling you how bad you feel, how tired you are, and trying to convince you to just give up and walk off the floor. That's your body. On the other shoulder, an angel encourages you, reminding you how much better you're going to feel if you just get through the next few reps. That's your spirit. Let's add a third character: your mind. Your mind is somewhere in the middle, sitting on the fence, listening to both sides of the story, trying to decide which way to go. Now, your mind can take either side, depending on what kind of information it has. You're going to take some action. Will it be positive or negative? Will you keep going or will you quit?

No matter how you feel, no matter what you know, in the end, it's your will that determines how you put those feelings and that knowledge into action. It's your will that makes it possible for you to put your faith into action, to make what you believe in happen for you. I always say that Knowledge is power. So as you reach that point where you're in danger of quitting, remember this:

- *Muscle fatigue is a goal of vigorous exercise, not a bad side effect.* Of course, you should never exercise in any way that's likely to cause injury or that feels unusual or painful to you. But burning muscles, tired muscles, muscles that shake a little when you hold a position for more than a few seconds—that's what you're working toward.

- *Muscle fatigue tells you that you're working out harder than you have before.* And that's a good thing.

- *Muscle fatigue is temporary.* No matter how tired your muscles feel, within minutes, even seconds of shifting to another activity, that heavy "I can't hold this one more second" feeling will disappear.

- *Muscle fatigue is necessary to build muscles, increase your endurance, and exercise that will.* If you never reached this point in your Workout, you'd never learn what it is to work your will in addition to your body. You wouldn't be doing Tae-Bo.

- *Muscle fatigue is a great test of your will.* Who's the boss? Who's the brains? You are! Don't let your body tell you what to do.

Manage Fatigue Before It Takes Control

There are ways to work around your fatigue. Here are the tricks that will help you keep working out when your muscles are telling you to sit down.

- *As you feel specific muscles fatigue, shift your movement temporarily to another muscle group.* To relieve some of the heaviness you may feel in your muscles, keep moving but move different body parts. So if your legs are getting hard to move, try throwing some punches. If your arms are giving you trouble, march or do some kicks. After eight counts, try to get back into the Workout.

- *When repetitions become difficult, try slowing down your pace and doing the same move in half time.* In other words, do in two beats what everyone else is doing in one. As soon as you can, resume the regular count.

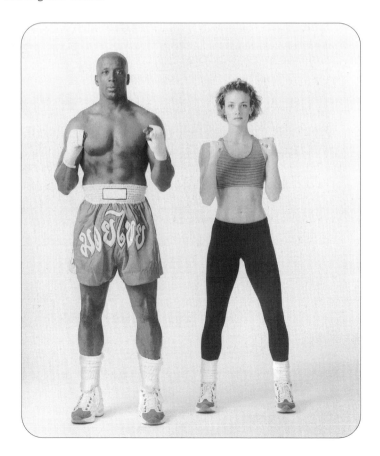

- *If you find yourself breathing hard, slow it down and concentrate on breathing more naturally.* Remember: Your body reacts to reaction. Your brain responds to what your ears hear. Not only does taking long, labored breaths slow you down, it can set off a surge of adrenaline that makes you feel nervous or panicky.

- *When you're doing legwork and your muscles start to feel heavy and tired, continue the same movement but change the muscles you're working by changing your foot position.* If you're flexing your foot, try a set with your toes pointed. If your toes are pointed, try a set with your foot flexed. The reason this works is that pointing your toe, generally, makes your leg feel lighter. It also works the muscles in the front of your leg, while a flexed foot works those at the back.

- *If your muscle fatigue is concentrated on one side or in a particular muscle, the cause could be poor technique.* Check yourself, correct your movements, and then continue. (See the "Troubleshooting Your Technique" chapter for more specific information.)

When You Should S T O P Your Workout

If you need to march in place or get a drink of water, do so, then come back. But you should stop your Workout immediately and call your doctor if you feel any of these symptoms:

- lightheadedness

- pain or heaviness in your chest, arm, shoulder, or jaw

- dizziness

- nausea

- unusually rapid or erratic heartbeat

- difficulty catching your breath

Your body's telling you it's time to take a rest.

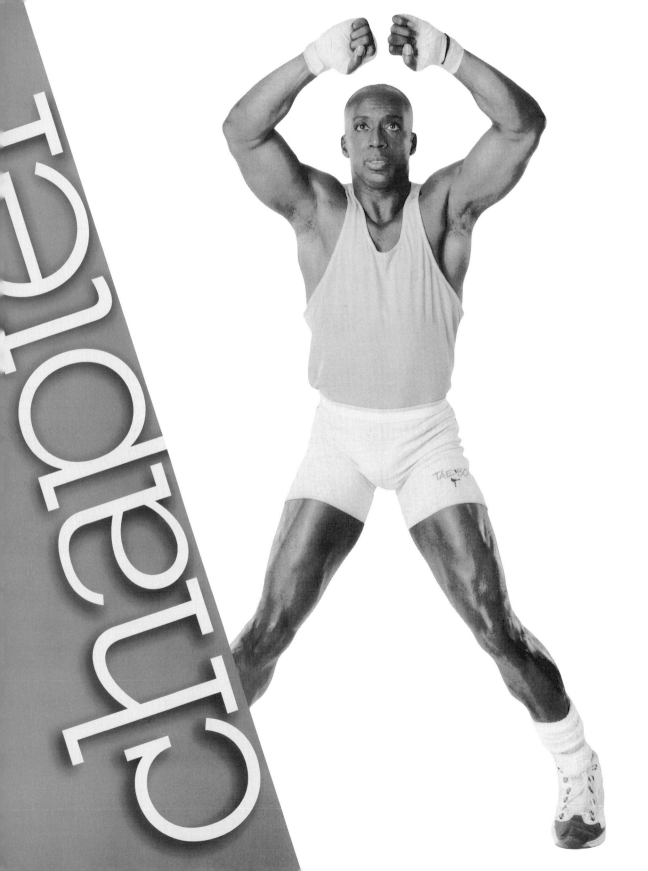

five

The Principles of Tae-Bo

Tae-Bo is easy to learn because even the most complex combinations can be broken down into a series of basic movements. The Basic Techniques are the foundation of your Workout. These are exactly the same moves I teach in classes and on the videotapes, and they are all the movements you need to know to master whatever new combinations and moves I develop and add to Tae-Bo in the years to come.

Even if you've been doing Tae-Bo for a while now, I encourage you to read this chapter carefully. It distills not only what I and other certified Tae-Bo instructors have been teaching, but also what we've learned from students. Know that if you've ever had trouble distinguishing a Roundhouse Kick from a Side Kick, or if the exact difference between a Hook and a Cross seems hard to pin down, you are not alone. In the photographs and the detailed instructions, I've tried to anticipate and answer your questions. (You can also consult "Troubleshooting Your Technique" in Chapter 8.) Yes, a picture is worth a thousand words, but be sure to read the accompanying pointers, especially the sections titled "Principles" and "What's Wrong with This Picture?" which are in Chapter 7.

If your awareness is high, it doesn't matter how low you kick.

First, Be an Observer

Before you do anything, always watch. Awareness is a pillar of Tae-Bo. Watch each videotape several times before you actually try to do the Workout and read through this section. Once you've started doing the Workout, remember that the more you learn and the more you do, the more you can learn and the more you can do.

One of the best things you can do is develop good habits in your Workout. It's easy to fall into the habit of not turning your standing foot out enough before a kick or raising your elbow an inch or two too high when you punch. That's why it's always a good idea to review the videotapes and this book even after you've mastered the techniques. That way you can spot and correct those bad habits before they take hold. And I guarantee, you'll always find something you can apply to make your Workout even better.

Now, after I've said so much about watching and reading and looking at the pictures, I want to warn you: Your eyes can deceive you, especially when you're watching yourself work out. No matter how carefully you study the tapes or this book, you won't truly be learning the Workout until your body begins learning it. And the body, unlike the mind, learns only through the experience of doing.

So how can your eyes deceive you? First, your eyes don't always see everything. You may be watching yourself in a mirror doing a kick, but even as you watch yourself, you have to remember that in executing the move, you're splitting your attention from carefully observing, and in observing yourself, you're probably not focusing completely on your movements. I believe it's better to learn a Basic Technique first without watching yourself. Practice it, talk it through to yourself, count out the steps, and keep your eyes on what you're doing. That means that you should always look in the direction that you're moving, kicking, or punching. Always hold that focus.

Once you feel comfortable with a move, try doing it with your eyes closed. If you're like most Tae-Bo students, you'll discover that your timing and your performance improve after a few "blind" reps. Why is this? Aside from the fact that watching yourself can be a little distracting, I think that closing your eyes and moving forces your mind to call on the visual picture inside your mind. When I tell my students to think of each movement as a print, what I mean is this: You want it to be clean and sharp, with no blurring around the edges. The original that you strike that fresh print from is inside your mind. It's what you see and then try to copy with every repetition. When you feel like you've mastered the basic aspects of a move, then turn to the mirror and use it to clean up the last few mistakes in your technique.

Practice, Remembering That You Are Your Own Coach

After that, mastering your Workout is a matter of practicing and striving for the best technique. Don't let yourself settle for anything short of the best you can do—whether you're barely sweating through that easy first twenty minutes or struggling through the fire, the trials and tribulations of working out. When you reach that point in Tae-Bo where you're calling on your will and drawing on your spirit, you don't want to say to yourself, "Step, pivot, knee raise, kick, foot down, weight shift. . . ." You want to know what you're doing and why. Then you want your movements to go beyond being something that you do with your body to being something that you feel with every part of you—body, mind, and spirit. When I say that Tae-Bo works from the inside out, that's what I mean.

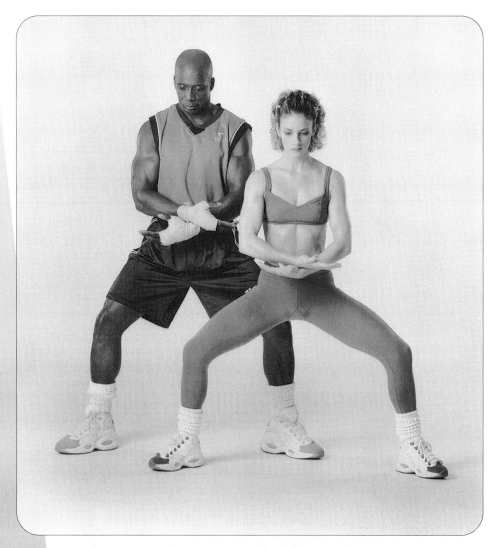

Always remember, your coach is inside you. You are the boss.
I can't count the times a student has said to me, "I'm doing the
Workout, but I know I'd do it better (or more often, or with clean-
er technique, or with a stronger commitment, or whatever) if I
could train with you personally." I always tell them that they're
wrong. That even if I stood an inch away from you and talked you
through every move you made, I am powerless to change anything about you or how you do your Workout. It's all inside you:
the will, the courage, the power. A hundred coaches could
stand around you twenty-four hours a day. But they couldn't
make you lift a finger if you didn't have the will to do it.

This is also why you need to hold in your mind a strong,
clear image of what you want your body to do. After you've

studied the videotapes and the book, your guide is going to be you. That's why you have to concentrate and keep your movements in sync with your thoughts. As I've explained before, this is what I mean when I tell you not to move between thoughts. Make every motion, no matter how small, have a definite beginning and a definite end. Use the Principles of Tae-Bo to help you pull it all together.

The Principles of Tae-Bo

As you know, every stance, step, knee raise, kick, punch, exercise, or combination requires thought and focus. The instructions in Chapter 7 will tell you how to do the moves, what to look out for, and how to spot mistakes. What follows here are the hidden instructions, the knowledge I and my instructors offer students in our classes. This is the information students pick up without even realizing it—by watching and listening to the hundreds of suggestions and corrections we offer every class. Since you may be working out alone, or with your family or a friend or two, without a certified Tae-Bo instructor looking over your shoulder, take some time to study these Principles. These outline the basic awareness you should bring to every Workout and every move. Whether you've been doing Tae-Bo for a while or are just beginning, keep these Principles fresh in your mind. Go back and look at them now and then. They'll help you to better understand the instructions that follow. And don't think that you're at a disadvantage just because you're not working out in a class with a teacher. Always remember that the real coach is inside you.

Always be aware—of your surroundings, of your movements, and of yourself.

It's not unusual for people—especially as they start to tire—to let their minds begin to wander. If you're working out and thinking about what to have for dinner tonight, stop and refocus. Keep yourself alert by thinking about what you're doing. Ask yourself, "How do I feel?"; "What made that punch feel so much smoother than the one I did a minute ago?"; "Why is this kick so low today?"; "Where do I feel it in my arm with the Jab? And where do I feel it with the Hook?" Use your Workout to know your body and become its master. Once you get into the habit of focusing, it will be harder to think about anything else.

Renew your thoughts.

When you renew your thoughts, you're doing much more than just adopting new ideas about your Workout or reminding yourself why you started in the first place. When I say you should renew your thoughts, I mean that you should take a moment each day to tell yourself not only what you've promised yourself you would do, but why. It's not always easy to stay inspired, but you can do it if you keep alive the positive feelings you have about your Workout. This is something that no one can do for you. Before every Workout, rededicate yourself to what you're about to do.

Always be ready to learn something new.

If you've learned to move in ways that are different from what we do in Tae-Bo, don't worry. Nothing that you may be doing is right or wrong. The exception is a movement that might create stress or injury, and we point those out throughout "The Basic Techniques" (Chapter 7) and "Troubleshooting Your Technique" (Chapter 8). I believe in Tae-Bo, but I don't believe that there's any exercise or activity that's right or wrong, better or worse. I never ask my students to forget anything they've ever learned or done before. Just give me the chance to show you how to do something in a different way.

Pace yourself.

You can go through the fire. Only you know your limitations, and these can change from one day to the next. Be aware of things that could be making your Workout harder (exhaustion, stress, illness, not eating well, and so on), and try to work around them today. Throughout the exercise instructions, I suggest tips for customizing your Workout so you can modify it through tough spots. You don't have to quit. You can shift your focus, your movements, and your energy and continue.

Breathe correctly.

No matter how hard you're working out, try to breathe as naturally as possible. That might mean breathing faster and harder, but it shouldn't mean stopping now and then to take huge, deep, gasping gulps of air. Also be aware of tensing up and not breathing whenever you're executing a demanding move or delivering a punch or a kick. If you come out of a move needing a really deep breath, chances are you weren't breathing well or at all during the move before that. Keep your breathing constant and in time to your Workout. Learn to inhale with every pulling motion and exhale with every pushing motion, and you should do fine. That means:

- Exhale at the point of impact of a punch or kick, and whenever you are concentrating on your upper-body muscles (for an abdominal crunch, for instance).
- Inhale on recovering your punch or kick, and whenever you return to the start position in any other move.

As you progress through Tae-Bo, breathing correctly will become second nature to you.

Learn to count music.

Depending on who you are, that probably sounds either very simple or very complicated. Even if you're the type who hasn't set foot on a dance floor in years, you can still do Tae-Bo. And it's not a question of having rhythm either. A sense of rhythm is really just the ability to count music correctly. Remember: Almost all popular music is written in measures of eight beats each. When you learn to count beats correctly, you'll find it much easier to stay in the rhythm of the Workout. You can practice by counting along as you listen to music and counting aloud as you work out.

Count out loud as you go.
Remember: Your body reacts to reaction.

You might think that counting out loud and counting silently to yourself are the same. They're not. Your body responds to sound, and you can test this yourself by trying a four-part combination—let's say, Left Jab, Right Cross, Left Jab, clap—while counting out loud and then repeating the combination while counting silently to yourself. Which combination moved better, felt stronger, and had more power? There's probably a deep psychological reason why voicing our intentions makes them easier to follow through. All I know is that in Tae-Bo, counting out loud as you work out improves your technique, increases your stamina, and almost guarantees that you're breathing correctly.

> *Don't waste your time trying to become "just like" someone else. Be the best that you are.*

Develop your sense of balance.

People often think that their sense of balance is something they're either born with or not. Balance—like any skill—can be improved through Tae-Bo, but first you may have to learn

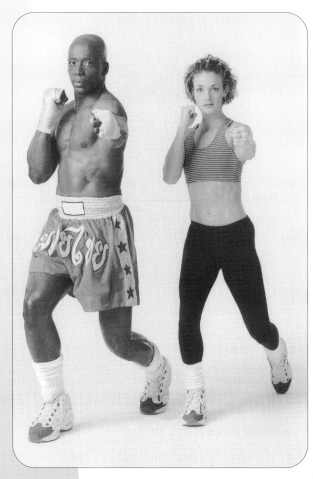

some new habits and unlearn some others. If the first image you think of when someone says "balance" is a tightrope walker with both arms extended outward from her body, forget it. The closer you can keep your arms to your body, the better you'll be able to balance. In Tae-Bo, if you find yourself losing your balance, try not to throw your arms out. Remember: The foundation of your balance is in the middle of your body. So if you are trying to balance on one leg, try moving up and down slightly on your bent leg instead of wobbling from side to side.

Even the position of your head—determined in part by which way you look—can affect your balance. So make sure you have a clear mental picture of where your move is going and a focus point for its destination, or point of impact. Keep your eyes trained on that point. Shifting your gaze from your feet to your hands to your legs to whatever else you see will throw you off balance. (For more on balance, see pages 130-131.)

Sharpen your sense of positioning.

First, realize that every day, your body is constantly performing movements that you don't even think about. In our daily lives, that's a good thing, because it allows us to focus on other things going on around us, like what the car ahead is doing or what someone is saying. But when you work out, you have to break the habit of moving automatically. You have to learn to move with more self-awareness. Let me give you a little test: Stand up and without looking at your feet or your legs, describe their position:

- Are you placing more weight on one leg?
- Or is it equally distributed between both?
- Which way are your toes pointed?
- Are your knees locked, or straight but relaxed, or bent?

There are no right or wrong answers here. But I'll bet you couldn't answer those questions without stopping to think about it and look. That's because we move without thinking all the time. I promise you, Tae-Bo will change how you move—and not just when you're working out. How does it happen? Two ways. First, you need to focus so intensely to learn and to execute Tae-Bo, you can't help but become more aware. Second, in continuing to do Tae-Bo and working through greater challenges, you sharpen your body consciousness even more.

FOCUS. You hear that word a lot, but here's what it means in my class: Pay attention to only one thing at a time.

That means when you're working out, imagine and visualize a target or opponent for every movement. Tae-Bo works on so many levels because it demands that you focus your concentration, your energy, and your strength. To direct and control your movement, you must have mental focus. Now think about throwing a punch out anywhere in the air. Without direction, you have no purpose. Without purpose, you have no focus. And without focus, you have no control. Now stop and think how much better that same punch would be if you had a clear, specific target. You wouldn't drive in a strange place without a map or send your children someplace without knowing why they were going there. It's human nature not to do things well when we don't know why we're doing them. Knowing where you're going and why makes all the difference in anything you do.

Focus on working each body part individually while at the same time making sure that every Tae-Bo move is executed with your full body.

It sounds like a contradiction, doesn't it? But think it through. Focusing on each body part as you move it keeps you from using your shoulders to support your arms or kicking from your knees instead of your hips. Making your Tae-Bo moves full-body moves means that your entire body is coiled and ready. It means that even though you're punching with a fist or kicking with a foot, you're putting the power of your whole body behind it. Remember: The part of your body you're moving is just the focal point of your entire body's energy and force.

Complete every move with full concentration and control at every stage.

The goal of a punch isn't that moment of impact but the correct execution of every stage of the movement, from the starting position to the recovery. In fact, it's often easier to punch out than it is to bring your fist back following the same pathway while positioning your whole body correctly for the next move. Failing to follow through with your movements not only compromises the benefit of your Workout, it increases your risk of injury.

Break down every move while you're learning it, then go for flow.

There's a lot going on in Tae-Bo, and it can take you a while to pull together all the elements that make a good kick, for instance. Breaking each move down and stopping to consciously think it through as you learn it is like using training wheels on your bike. It may not look too smooth, but it's necessary. Once you have the technique down, though, try to think less about what you're doing and focus instead on the purpose of each move, the role each of your body parts is playing, and your target. Let the actual movements become as natural to you as riding a bike without training wheels.

Learn and apply the ways of reciprocal force.

You don't need a degree in physics to understand how and why a movement that uses both pushing and pulling muscles simultaneously is effective. The difference between executing a move and recovering to the start position is in which muscles are working at a particular instant. Take a punch. Delivering the punch may look like it's all push, but your pulling muscles are what keep the punch in control and stop you from extending your arm fully. Then at the moment of impact—not before or after—your pulling muscles are taking charge, bringing that fist back toward you in a carefully controlled movement. In addition to ensuring good technique, reciprocal force creates momentum that helps your muscles move efficiently, gives you a little jump of energy going into the next move, and keeps your body locked into a groove. Learning to use reciprocal force is the key to developing real flow.

Make sure to move through the full range of motion each and every time.

Once you get a little tired, it's natural to try and save some energy by limiting your movement. And you may notice that you're not punching or kicking as fully as you would if you weren't starting to feel fatigued. But thinking that you can save up your energy and your strength by holding back will work against you. Limiting your movement does not really save your energy. It also seriously compromises your Workout and—worst of all—sets you up for possible injury.

Let's look at what happens in a compromised punch. Instead of delivering a punch from the right position with a firm, correct fist, extending your arm two or three inches short of full extension, and then fully recovering your arm, you just carelessly push your hand out a few inches, then let it drop back to your side. Because you're not using reciprocal force to your advantage, the next punch is actually going to be harder to execute because you don't have that springlike momentum going for you. You may not notice it right away, but what you're sure to feel within the next few minutes is a gnawing cramp in your neck, your shoulder, or your upper back, because every time you restrict motion, you constrict your muscles. Just try this: Throw one full, completed punch, then try one with a floppy fist that goes out a few inches and then drops. The "easy" one is actually harder to do and harder on your body. If you feel that you absolutely cannot do three sets of eight full punches, do as many as you can correctly, then march in place until the next move.

Acknowledge and work on your weak spots.

We each have one side that is stronger than the other. Chances are, if you're right-handed, the left side of your body is not as strong as your right. You'll notice that I start most exercises on the left side. That's because most people are right-handed. If you happen to be left-handed and your left side is stronger, start on the right instead. I always like to work the weaker side first because most people have to put a little more concentration and effort into learning and then executing a move on that side. Starting on the weaker side lets you work that side fresh, before you tire.

Take a few minutes each time you do Tae-Bo to concentrate on working your weak side with an extra twenty-four kicks or punches. You might try doing this to any music you happen to like, since that will also help sharpen your sense of rhythm and your ability to keep the count. You might also discover that there are some Tae-Bo moves that come more naturally to you than others. For example, women are usually stronger in the lower body, while men usually have a stronger upper body.

Or you may have to apply some extra effort to those moves that depend on muscles that need work. For most people, that would be their abdominals. Always remember, though: You don't need great abs to do Tae-Bo, but if you keep doing Tae-Bo, you'll get them.

Set goals that are consistent with Tae-Bo.

People often come to physical fitness with a goal-oriented attitude. Having goals is great, but you have to define those goals very carefully. It's one thing to work toward the goal of doing forty Roundhouse Kicks each day. It's another thing to work toward doing each of those forty Roundhouse Kicks completely without cutting any corners on your technique. Almost anyone can kick forty times. But only a few can do that while maintaining the right position, keeping their balance, and returning fully to the starting Horse Stance each and every time.

Go for the flow.

Think of your Workout as one flowing series of movements. For me, the image of Tae-Bo at its best is movement with the precision and power of a machine *and* the flexibility and flow of water. To many people, those two images would seem opposite, and they are. The beauty of Tae-Bo is that your Workout can include both. When you start a movement with your feet, knees, and legs in the correct position, you can redirect the energy of your last movement into the next. That momentum sets the rhythm that locks your Workout into a groove. And always keep moving.

Work at your own pace.

There is a correct form to every Tae-Bo stance and move. However, no two people are exactly the same. When you study the videotapes, you'll notice slight differences in how each of us positions our body or executes a move. As you study these positions, experiment with how deeply you bend your knee and the position of your foot. Find the place where you can achieve good technique *and* hold your balance. If you feel yourself losing balance as you lower into the Horse Stance, for instance, don't go so low for now. If it's easier for you to pivot with your feet a few inches wider than shoulder-distance apart, then do so. Just always be aware that anytime you compromise in your technique, you may not be getting as much out of that exercise as you could. Perfect form in every movement is not possible for everyone doing Tae-

Bo. And it shouldn't prevent you from doing the Workout. But it should remain a constant goal—an idea of what you are working toward. Don't let what you can't do today keep you from working toward what you might achieve tomorrow. You never truly know how much better you can be.

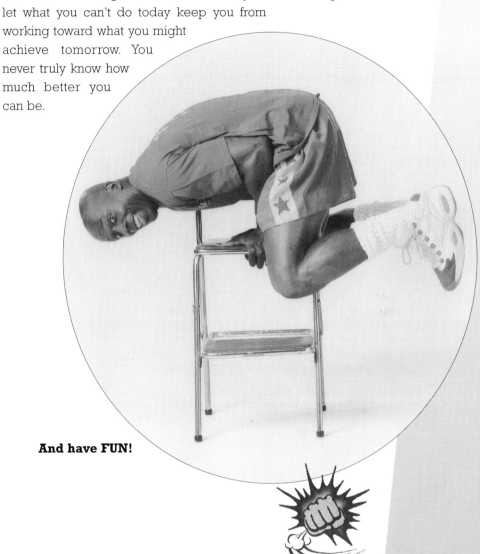

And have FUN!

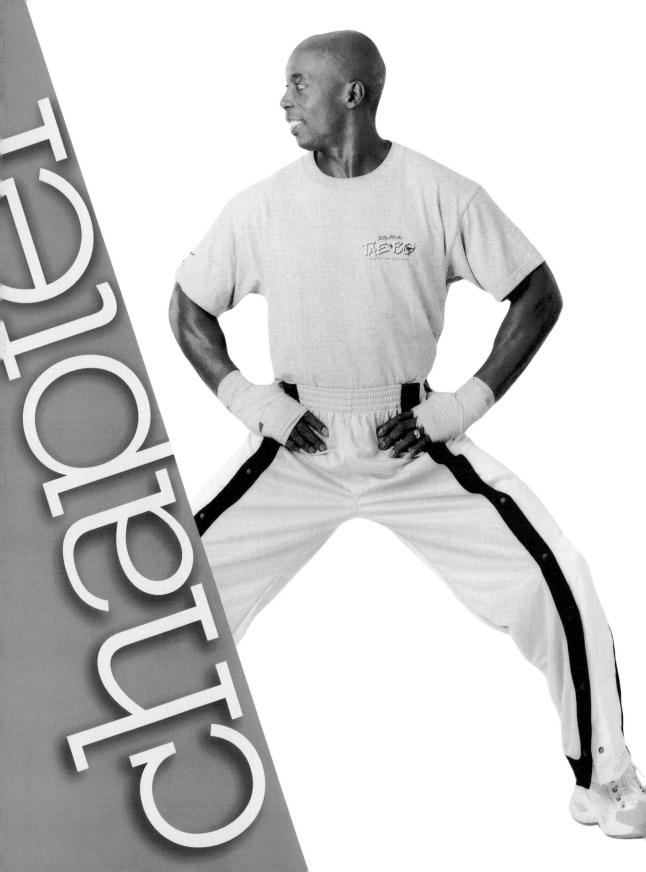

SIX

The Warm-Up

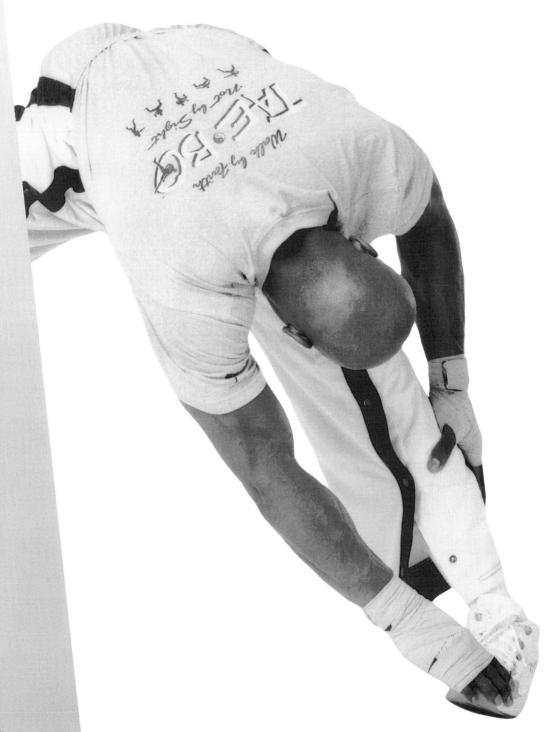

The first rule to remember about the Warm-up is that you should never work out without it. You may be short of time, anxious to get to the real Workout, or just feeling like you don't need it, but, believe me, you do. Everyone needs to warm up before working out—even if you are just learning or practicing the basic Tae-Bo techniques.

In many ways, the Warm-up is more important than the Workout itself, because the success of your Workout—and your ability to avoid injury—depend on it. The reason is simple: Warm muscles are more flexible, more agile, more responsive, and stronger. Warming up gives your heart the chance to start picking up the pace and gives your muscles a greater supply of blood and oxygen. A good Warm-up prepares you for the Workout and leaves you ready to react instantly. When you work out without warming up, you may find yourself struggling through the movements and becoming fatigued as you try to push yourself to do things your body just isn't ready or prepared to do.

Your Warm-up should be focused, smooth, and done slowly enough to be thorough. How long you spend warming up depends on how you feel. Generally, you should spend at least five to seven minutes. You can also do extra sets for specific areas; for example, if your neck is especially tight, or if your hamstrings don't seem to be stretching as easily as usual.

Also, use your Warm-up to renew the connection between your mind and your body. As you go through the Warm-up exercises, focus on what you're doing and how you're feeling. If anything feels tight, give it a few more minutes of slow stretching and movement until it feels right to you. Check in on yourself: How does each movement feel? What feels easier today than it did yesterday? What do you want to get out of your Workout today?

The Tae-Bo Warm-up works from the head right down to the toes. As you warm up, remember to control each movement. Breathe naturally, and be especially careful not to hold your breath when you're stretching. Visualize what you're doing and what you're trying to achieve. Feel your heart rate start to rise and your muscles start to warm up. Use the time to put all of your thoughts aside and really concentrate on the Workout ahead. Maybe today you're going to get through the Workout without stopping, or add extra sets to your Floor Work, or kick an inch or two higher. Whatever it is, talk to yourself. And don't tell yourself you're going to "try." Tell yourself that you're going to "do."

When you reach the end of the Warm-up, rise slowly and carefully, take a deep breath, and you'll be ready to go.

THE WARM-UP

Do each of the stretches throughout the Warm-up for one or two sets of eight counts. Never do fewer repetitions than suggested, and do more if you feel you need to.

1 Start in a Forward Stance, with your hands on your hips.

2 Step to the side—first with your right foot and then with your left—until your feet are about six inches wider than shoulder-width apart. Relax your knees so that both are slightly bent.

3 While keeping your back straight, squat into a semi-sitting position. Bend your knees, but not beyond the point where you can't see your toes. Also bend at the hip joints (*not* at the waist). Keep your back straight, your abs tight, and rest your hands loosely on your hips. (This is a variation of the Horse Stance.)

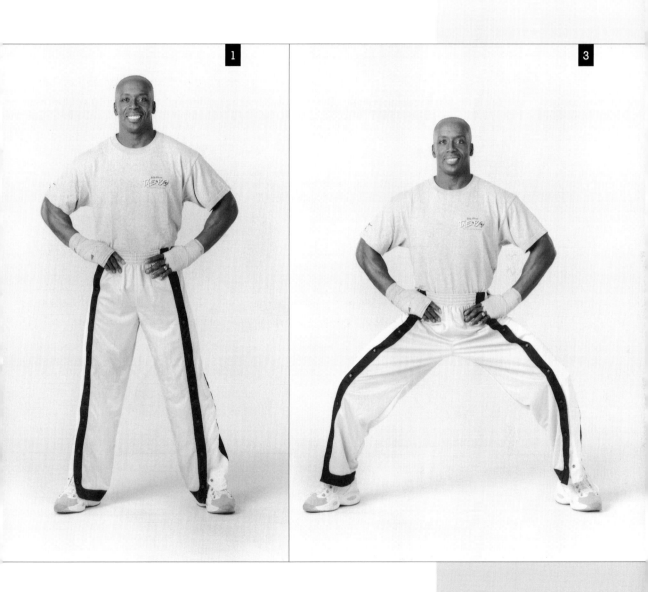

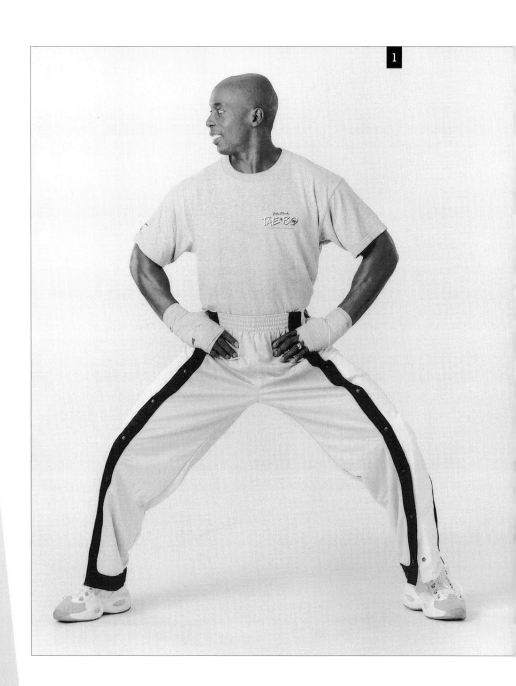

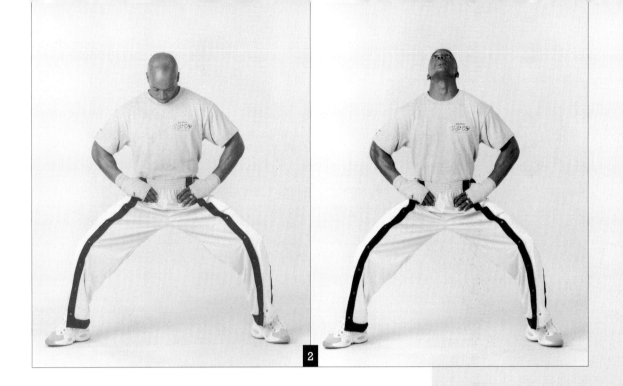

2

WARM UP THE NECK

These moves stretch and relax the neck muscles, an area where many of us accumulate muscle tension. As you work your neck muscles, remember to keep your movements slow and flowing. Avoid sudden, jerky motions, and never rotate your neck in a full circle. Breathe naturally throughout. Each movement is done in one count. In other words, "right" equals "one," "left" equals "two." Do two to three sets of 8 reps.

1 Standing tall with your chin parallel to your shoulders, turn your head first to the right and then to the left. Look in the direction that you're turning and focus on stretching the neck muscles as you move. Do two to three sets of 8 reps.

2 Next, stretch your neck forward by bringing your chin down toward your chest, up through the start position, and back. As you stretch back, concentrate on stretching your neck upward as well so your neck doesn't curve forward and your head doesn't just drop back. Remember to control the motion all the way through. Do two to three sets of 8 reps.

WARM UP THE ARMS
AND UPPER BODY

Here again, the emphasis should be on stretching. This is a good stretch for your upper body, but you should feel it especially in your back, arms, and sides. Try not to bounce or jerk as you change direction. Focus on the alignment of your body. When you're bending to the side, go straight to the side without leaning forward or back.

1 Still in the Horse Stance, bring your left hand over your head and your right hand across your lower body.

2 Without bending very much at the waist, concentrate on using your left arm to stretch your upper body. Stretch for a count of 8.

3 Change sides, bringing your right hand over your head and your left hand across your lower body. Stretch for a count of 8.

4 From the Horse Stance, raise your left arm to shoulder level and extend it fully in front of you. At the same time, pivot both feet to the right and reach to the right. Use your whole body to pivot. Focus on stretching the muscles in your waist and back. Stretch for a count of 8.

5 Return to the starting Horse Stance. Raise your right arm to shoulder level and extend it fully in front of you. At the same time, pivot both feet to the left and reach to the left. Use your whole body to pivot. Focus on stretching the muscles in your waist and back. Stretch for a count of 8.

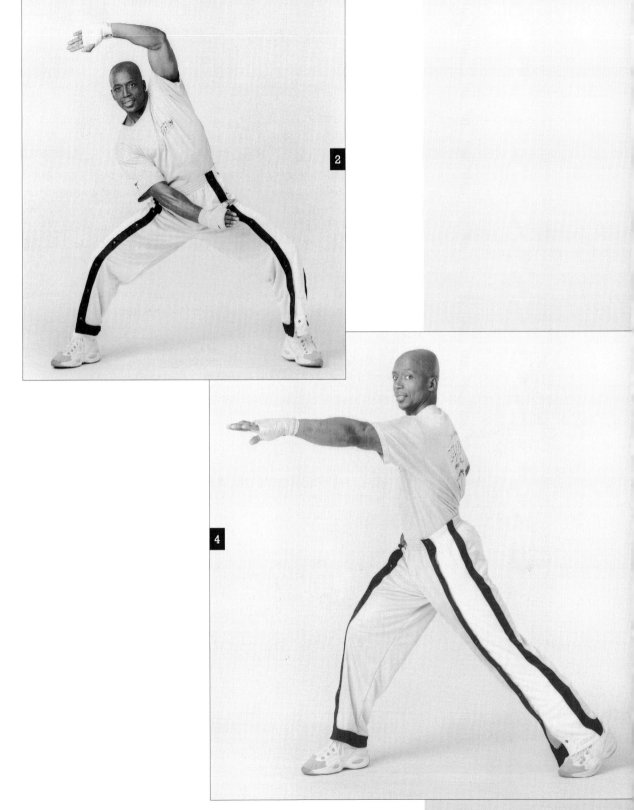

2

4

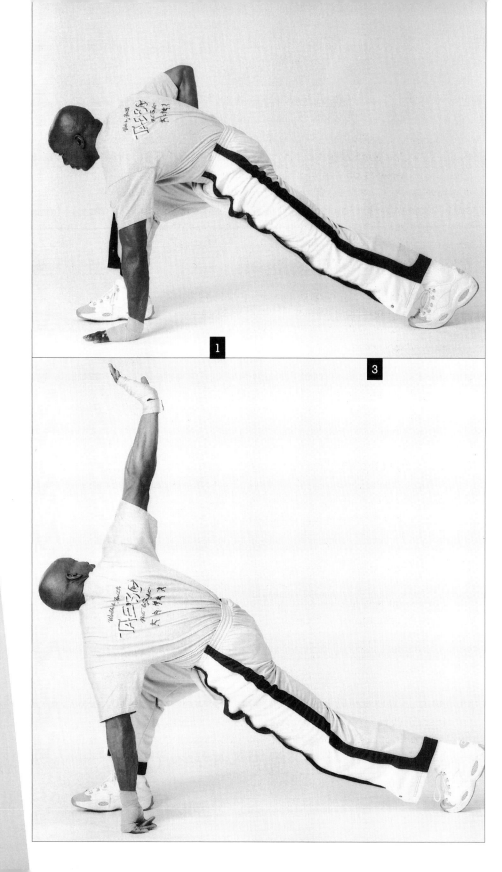

WARM UP THE LEGS

When you're working on your legs during the Warm-up, you want to be sure that you're really stretching carefully and thoroughly. While the focus is on the legs, try to think about stretching the muscles in your neck and your back. Consciously relaxing your neck and back muscles will help you stretch forward more easily. Whenever you bend, breathe out. When you stretch up, breathe in. Never do a kick before your leg muscles are completely warmed up.

1 From the starting Horse Stance, pivot with both feet and lunge to the right, placing your left palm on the floor beside your right foot. (Please see page 108 for pointers on pivoting correctly.)

2 Be sure that your right knee is bent but not covering your toes. Your left leg is fully extended with your left heel up off the floor and the weight on that side concentrated in the ball of your foot.

3 Twisting at the waist so that you're looking over your right shoulder, raise your right arm and extend it so your right palm is facing the ceiling. As you do this, focus on stretching the leg muscles—especially the hamstrings—of the left leg. Hold for a count of 8.

4 Lower your right arm and place both palms on the floor. As you do this, pivot back so both feet are facing forward and your legs are straight. Walk your hands to the center in front of you, then continue across to your left.

5 Pivot with both feet and lunge to the left, placing your right palm on the floor beside your left foot.

6 Be sure that your left knee is bent but not covering your toes. Your right leg is fully extended with your right heel up off the floor and the weight on that side concentrated in the ball of your foot.

WARM UP THE LEGS Continued

7 Twisting at the waist so that you're looking over your left shoulder, raise your left arm and extend it so your left palm is facing the ceiling. As you do this, focus on stretching the leg muscles—especially the hamstrings—of the right leg. Hold for a count of 8.

8 Lower your left arm and place both palms on the floor. As you do this, pivot back so both feet are facing forward and your legs are straight. Walk your hands to the center in front of you for the Standing Straddle Stretch.

9 Grab your left ankle with your left hand, your right ankle with your right. If you can't do this comfortably, place your hands on your calves or your knees.

10 For a count of 8, stretch down and back. Push your muscles gently. Don't bounce hard up and down.

11 Without lifting your head, bend over your left thigh and stretch for a count of 8.

12 Without lifting your head, move back to the middle, then to your right. Bend over your right thigh and stretch for a count of 8.

13 Slowly rise by first moving to the middle and uncoiling your back, starting from your lower back and straightening up vertebrae by vertebrae.

Take a breath.

WARM UP YOUR MIND

Concentrate your thoughts. Think how blessed you are to be here today. Take a moment to push back any distracting thoughts and recommit your energy to the Workout ahead. Remind yourself of everything you've achieved so far through your Workout, and use that to inspire you through whatever trials and tribulations may come your way today. Think about what you want to achieve today, then take a good, full breath, smile, and move into position. You're ready to go.

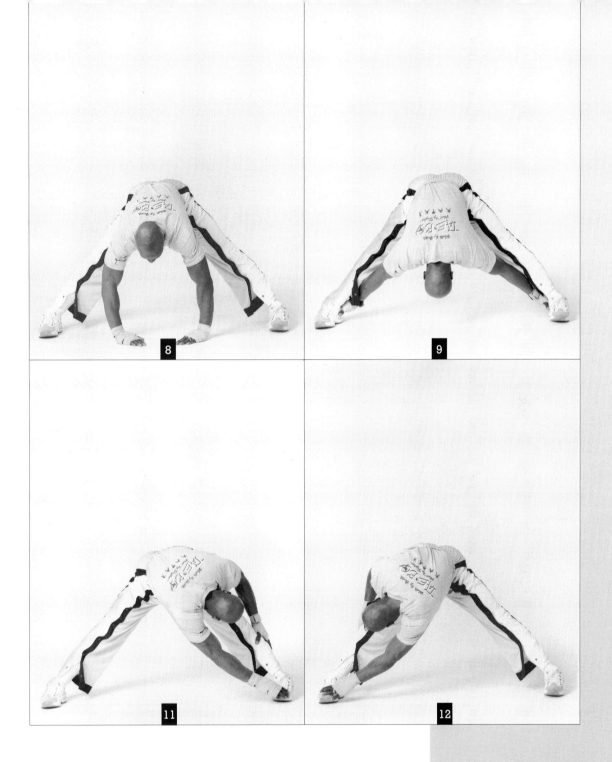

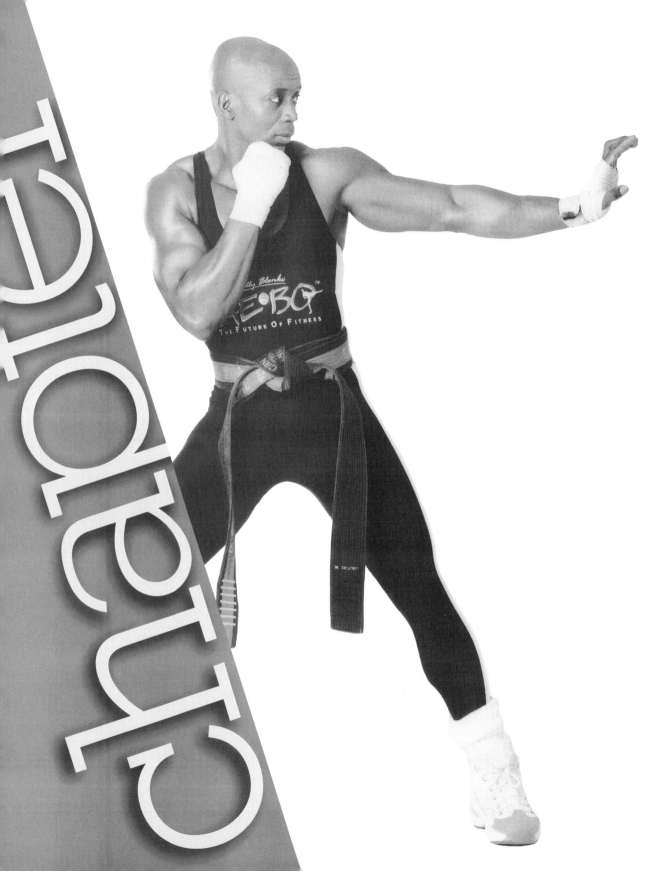

chapter

seven

The Basic Techniques

The Basic Techniques

Every Tae-Bo stance and move has a correct form. However, I also know that no two people are exactly the same. On the videotapes, you'll notice slight differences in how Shellie and I position our bodies or execute a move. We are each certified Tae-Bo instructors, and we know from experience what works for us. Soon you will know your own body just as well. As you study these positions, experiment with finding the position that's technically correct and the most comfortable for you. I want you to find the place where you can achieve good technique and hold your balance. If you feel yourself losing balance as you lower into the Horse Stance, for instance, don't go so low for now. If it's easier for you to pivot with your feet a few inches wider than shoulder-distance apart, then do so. If you can't kick as high as we do in the photographs, that's okay. Kick as high as you comfortably can, reminding yourself that a well-executed but lower kick is a step toward that higher kick.

However you have to modify your technique, always be sure that you're using your full range of motion. There's a difference between executing a perfect Front Kick that goes only as high as your knee (which is fine) and letting your fist flop and your arm drop in a Jab (which can result in discomfort or injury). Even when you're being careful about your modifications, always be aware that any time you compromise in your technique, you may not be getting as much out of that exercise as you could.

Perfect form in every movement is not possible for everyone doing Tae-Bo. And it shouldn't prevent you from doing the Workout. But it should remain a constant goal, what you are working toward. Don't let what you can't do today keep you from working toward what you might achieve tomorrow. You never truly know how much better you can be.

In the pages that follow, you'll find step-by-step instructions on all the Basic Techniques of Tae-Bo. Every movement and exercise is carefully illustrated with photographs that show you from several different angles what proper technique looks like and text that explains how to achieve it. Here you'll find the inside tips, pointers, and background information to help you truly understand the movements instead of just copying them. There's information on how to check your technique, how to modify your Workout to make it more or less challenging, and some insight into what you should be thinking and visualizing as you work out. And don't overlook "What's Wrong with This Picture?," a guide to poor technique and common mistakes.

the Stances

Every punch, every kick, and every combination in Tae-Bo begins from one of the following stances or from a minor variation on one of them. With practice and focus, you will be able to assume a stance as quickly and as easily as taking a step. When done correctly, a good stance works your thighs, hamstrings, lower stomach muscles, and lower back muscles. The Horse Stance is especially good for working the thighs and eliminating saddlebags.

The correct stance gives you the balance that is the foundation for everything we do in Tae-Bo. When you feel balanced, you have a keener sense of your physical center and a clear sense of the direction of your movements. This is important because as you move in Tae-Bo, you should always be visualizing the destination of your kick or your punch.

No degree of technical skill, no amount of physical strength can save a move that begins out of balance. And good balance starts with a steady stance. Once you find the correct position, you'll be able to shift your weight easily and get the sense of continual motion that makes Tae-Bo so enjoyable. The correct positions increase your accuracy and give your combinations and repetitions confidence, power, and flow.

For Every Stance, Remember:

Even when you're standing still in Tae-Bo, you are always poised and ready to move. Think like a snake. A snake that's lying perfectly straight and fully relaxed can't do anything. But a snake that's coiled, alert, aware, and slightly tensed is ready to strike on a second's notice. That's how I want you to be: always ready. Without tensing up your muscles, teach yourself to find a comfortable level of tension that lets you respond instantly. You'll know you've found it because when you get into your stance and bring your guard up, I promise, you will feel swifter and stronger. You'll find yourself thinking, "I *can* protect myself." And that's how you need to think to do Tae-Bo and to be a conqueror.

The Principles of Stances

These are the elements of your stance that apply for every position. At first, you may have to remind yourself and check yourself to be sure you're doing everything right. After a while, though, these will all become good habits that come naturally.

- Stand straight and face in the correct direction for your stance or movement. Keep your chin up, neck straight, shoulders back, and chest up. Visualize your rib cage suspended over your abdomen, not resting on it. Notice how much lighter and agile you feel, and how much more easily you can breathe.

- Always keep your abdominal muscles tight and firm. Think of these muscles as your center, the crossroads where your upper body and lower body meet. Developing strong abdominal muscles is one of the smartest investments you can make in your future health. Many back, hip, knee, and other joint-related problems are caused or made worse by weak abs.

- Learn to automatically bring your arms into a defensive guard position, no matter what your stance. That means your arms are bent at the elbow, with your fists held just under your chin, about four inches apart. Concentrate on holding your upper arms and elbows at your sides. Imagine each elbow tied to a rib; that's how close it should be. Usually, one fist will lead. It can be the punching fist or the fist on the side of your leading, or front, foot.

- Keep your arms close to your body in the guard position that's right for your stance or move. Remember: Balance lies at your center. The farther from your center you hold your arms, the less balanced you'll be.

- Pay attention to your feet and your knees. Even when you're standing with your legs straight, your knees should never lock and your feet should never rest flat with your weight focused on your heels. That's what I call a dead leg. Instead, keep the knees relaxed but ready to move, and your weight forward, on the ball of your foot, not the heel and not the toes. When you shift your weight back to the heel, don't do it out of habit. Do it with a clear purpose—to push off and throw some weight behind a punch or to stabilize a supporting leg for a kick.

- When you move into a stance, remember that you're not just positioning your various body parts. You're also aligning and distributing your weight—sometimes several times in a single move or combination. This is how you get maximum stability and power. Remember:

    Stationary weight provides stability.

    Weight in motion creates force.

So when you're kicking, you maintain balance by shifting most of your weight to the still, supporting leg. And when you're punching, you achieve force by shifting most of your weight behind your punching arm and your leading leg.

- If you're having trouble finding your balance, try to remain steady and centered. Instead of moving your body sideways to find your balance, try moving slightly up or down on your bent, supporting leg.

- Be aware. Listen and watch throughout the Workout. You will find that there are techniques—such as the Front Knee Raise, for instance—that begin with a Forward Stance with a slight change in positioning or a minor variation.

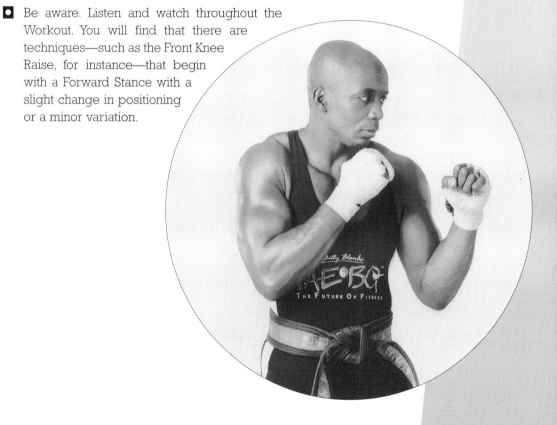

THE FORWARD STANCE

The Forward Stance—and the Left Side Stance and the Right Side Stance—help you keep your center of gravity high and stable. This gives your punches and your kicks power. It also makes it easy to move through combinations.

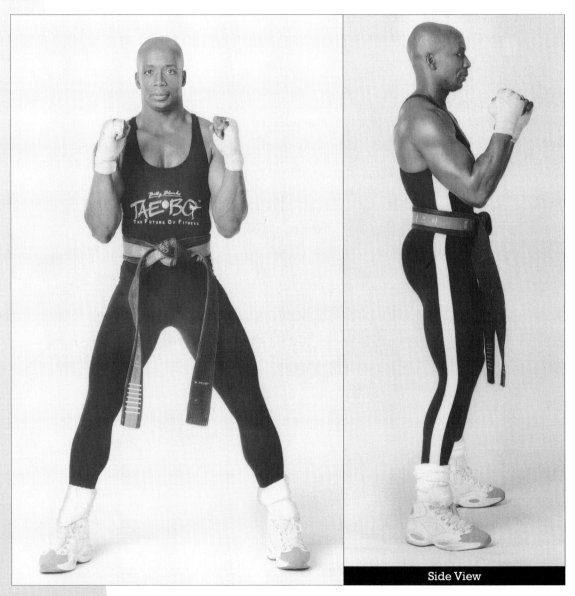

Side View

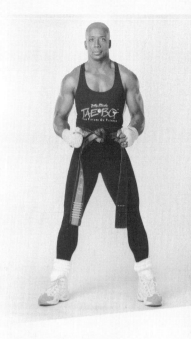

1 Stand facing forward with your feet parallel and about shoulder-width apart.

2 Bring your arms up into the guard position: With your upper arms and elbows resting tightly against your rib cage, bend your arms, so your fists are at chin height, aligned with your shoulder joint.

3 Keeping your left foot stable, step to your right with your right foot until your feet are a little wider than shoulder-distance apart. As you step, lift your foot decisively; don't let it glide or drag across the floor.

4 Your weight should be evenly distributed—50-50 on each foot—and focused on the balls of your feet, not on your heels.

5 Check your position: Your chin is up, your abs are tight, and your knees are slightly bent but not covering your toes.

What's Wrong with This Picture?

The Forward Stance

X My entire body is too relaxed. If you compare this picture to the others, you can tell that even my abs aren't as tight. I'm not ready to react.

X My guard is down. Even though my arms are bent, they're just hanging and pulling on my shoulders and rib cage. They feel heavier and harder to move.

X My legs are perfectly straight and my knees are locked instead of being slightly bent. It would be very difficult for me to move quickly in any direction from this position.

THE SIDE STANCES

Both Side Stances start from the Forward Stance. You move into position by stepping back with one foot, not forward. In both the Left Side Stance and the Right Side Stance, you begin with your weight distributed evenly between both legs. But to unlock the Side Stance's potential, you have to be ready to shift your weight to your front, or lead, leg. To make this easier, always:

- ❑ *keep the knees slightly bent and your back heel up*
- ❑ *keep your guard up, with your fists close together under your chin. In the Left Side Stance, your left fist should be four to six inches in front of your right. In the Right Side Stance, your right fist should be four to six inches in front of your left.*

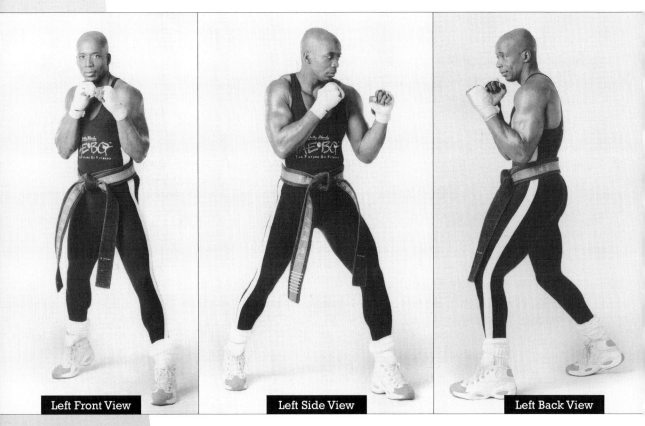

Left Front View   Left Side View   Left Back View

The Left Side Stance

1 From the Forward Stance, with your right foot, step about a shoulder-width back.

2 Your toes should be pointing straight ahead, and your feet should still be parallel—though not side by side.

3 Your weight should be evenly distributed between both legs. Your knees should be slightly bent and your right heel should be up off the floor, with the weight of that foot concentrated in the ball of your foot.

4 Your left fist should be four to six inches in front of your right fist.

The Right Side Stance

1 From the Forward Stance, with your left foot, step about a shoulder-width back.

2 Your toes should be pointing straight ahead, and your feet should still be parallel—though not side by side.

3 Your weight should be evenly distributed between both legs. Your knees should be slightly bent and your left heel should be up off the floor, with the weight of that foot concentrated in the ball of your foot.

4 Your right fist should be four to six inches in front of your left fist.

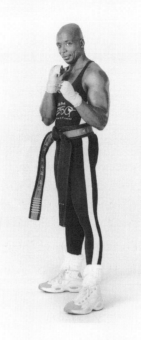

What's Wrong with This Picture?

The Side Stance

X *My legs are relaxed and my knees are straight instead of being slightly bent and ready to move. Even though my arms are bent and my hands are up, this is not a good guard. My hands are too far below my chin.*

X *My general body posture is weak. I'm standing on my heels and my abs aren't tight.*

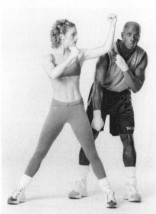

X *Shellie's feet are flat, her knees are locked, and her arms are not in a good guard position.*

X *Shellie's legs are too far apart, they are parallel, and her knees are locked, making her position very unstable.*

X *Her left fist is too high and too far away from her right. Her hands are too high to protect her.*

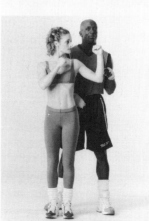

X *Shellie's feet are too close together and parallel. Also, her knees are locked, so it will be hard for her to move.*

X *There's too much distance between her fists for this to be a protective guard.*

THE HORSE STANCE

This classic martial-arts stance stabilizes your body by distributing most of your weight to your legs equally and lowering your center of gravity. The lower your center of gravity, the greater your stability. When you're in a Horse Stance, place your weight on your heels. Imagine that you're using your heels to grip the floor.

A well-executed Horse Stance is something you should really feel in your upper thigh muscles, your glutes, and your hamstrings. With practice, finding the correct position comes naturally.

Depending on what is most comfortable for you, your toes can either point forward or be slightly turned out.

1 From the Forward Stance, step to the side—first with your right foot and then with your left—until your feet are about six inches wider than shoulder-width apart.

2 Relax your knees so both are slightly bent.

3 While keeping your back straight, squat into a semi-sitting position. Bend your knees, but not beyond the point where you can't see your toes. Also, bend at the hip joints (*not* at the waist). Keep your back straight, your abs tight, and your arms up in guard position. Your upper arm and your elbows should be resting firmly against your rib cage.

As you master this technique, make sure to:

- Place most of your weight in your heels. Concentrating it in your toes puts too much pressure on your knees.

- Use your upper legs to sit into the position, with your weight focused in your heels and evenly distributed between both legs.

- Keep a strong, straight back. Don't thrust your pelvis forward, because it puts too much pressure on your knees. Some people do this without thinking, because they're trying to hold their backside in.

- As you move into the Horse Stance, remember that the aim here is a strong, balanced stance, not the lowest position you can reach. At first, you may not get as low as you would like. As long as your technique is good, that's okay. With time and practice, you'll be able to work comfortably from a lower position. If you look down at your knee and can't see your toes, there's too much stress on your knees.

- As you lower your body, visualize moving it straight down. Don't lower your butt by pushing it back and out behind you.

- In your deepest squat, your knee should be bent so the back of your thigh and the back of your lower leg form a 90-degree angle. If your butt is lower than your bent knees, your squat is far too deep, and you're risking injury.

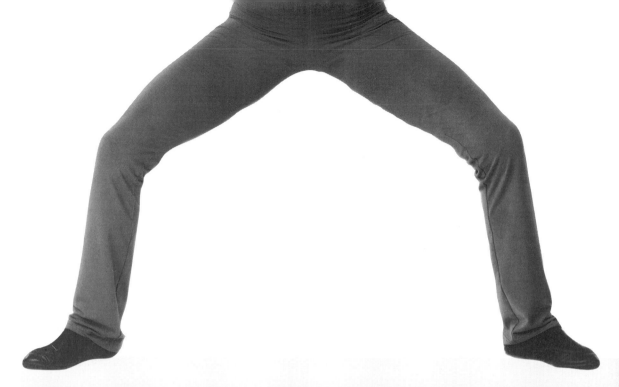

How to Master the Horse Stance

The Horse Stance is an exercise in itself. I urge you to practice wherever and whenever you can. I tell my students, Your body is the vehicle that has to carry you through this life. So it's important to keep the muscles of those tires—your legs and your knees—flexible and strong. Nothing builds strength and agility more quickly than the Horse Stance. Several times a day, whenever you have a few minutes—while you're talking on the phone, watching television, standing at your desk—drop into it. Work toward increasing the length of time you maintain it and shifting your body weight even lower down. You really want to feel the burn of your muscles working like they've never worked before. Believe me, after a few weeks, you'll see a big difference in your strength and stamina, not only during the Tae-Bo Workout but in everything else you do.

To make your Horse Stance more challenging:

▶ hold the Horse Stance you're doing now for extra counts, increasing the number every day

▶ hold the Horse Stance for the same number of counts you're doing now, but try to go down deeper in your squat

▶ do both: squat deeper for more counts (but do not squat beyond the point where your butt is lower than your knees)

To make it possible for you to hold your Horse Stance longer:

▶ find the point in your squat where you feel your muscles working without fatiguing too quickly

THE SIDE HORSE STANCE

The Side Horse Stance is the starting position for several Tae-Bo moves, including the Side Kick and the Roundhouse Kick. When you start Tae-Bo, you may think that the Side Horse Stance looks like a Side Stance, but there are some crucial differences.

- *You begin with your weight evenly distributed between your legs and centered in your heels. This gives you a strong foundation.*

- *Though your body faces forward, your head is turned to the right or the left, depending on the direction you're going to kick, punch, or move. Because you are not facing your imaginary opponent, you are vulnerable only on the lead side, and that's protected by your punch or kick. Even if you never spar with anyone, keep this information in mind, because it will help you maintain the correct position, especially when you're executing the Side Kick or the Roundhouse Kick.*

The Left Horse Stance

1 Start from the Horse Stance, facing forward.

2 Keeping your hips and shoulders facing forward, turn your head to face left.

3 Place your hands up, in guard position, with your left hand slightly higher than your right and a few inches farther out from your face than the usual guard position.

The Right Horse Stance

1 Start from the Horse Stance, facing forward.

2 Keeping your hips and shoulders facing forward, turn your head to face right.

3 Place your hands up, in guard position, with your right hand slightly higher than your left and a few inches farther out from your face than the usual guard position.

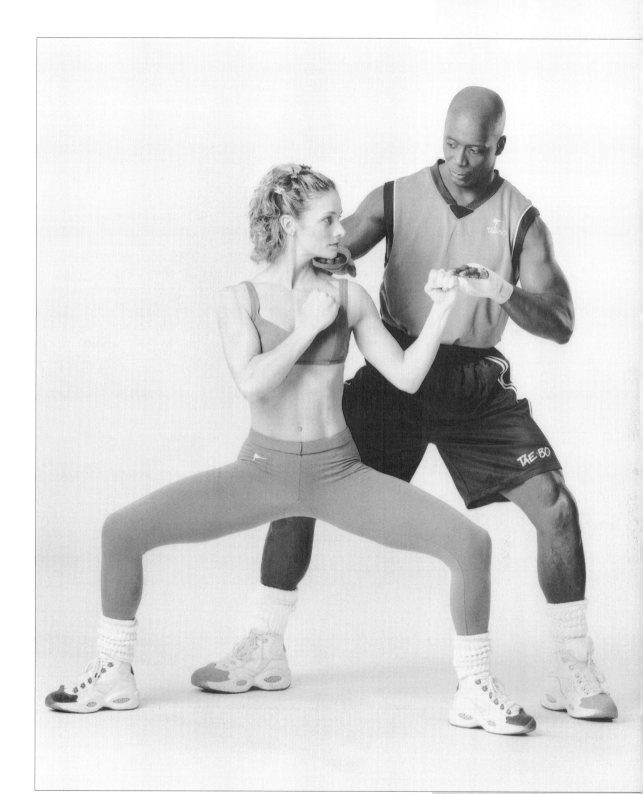

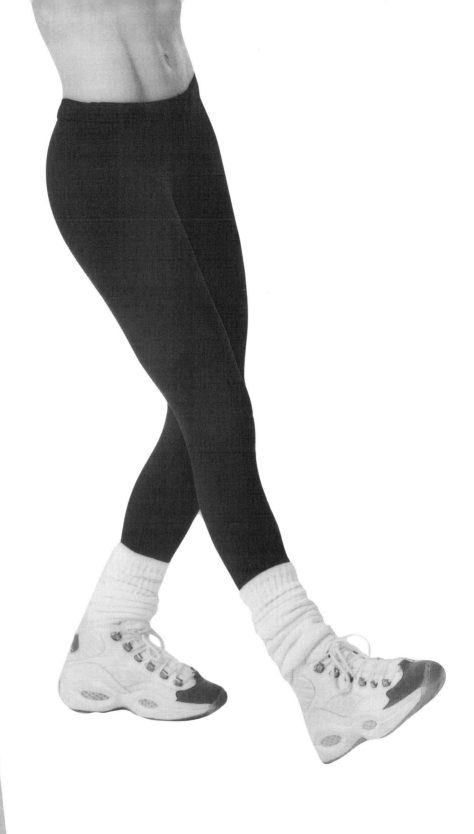

There isn't a lot of fancy footwork to Tae-Bo, but what we do use is very important. Tae-Bo is a whole-body workout, and every movement in your Workout begins from the ground up. I always tell students that how your feet move will determine how your whole body moves. Even when you are standing still in the Horse Stance, the part of the foot you're standing on will influence your speed, your agility, your reach, and your ability to react.

Just by watching you walk across a room, I can tell how you're going to move in Tae-Bo. If your feet drag as every part of your foot hits the floor almost simultaneously, your whole body is going to drag, no matter what you do. Besides, when you drag your foot, you create tension in your knees, which can lead to injury. If, on the other hand, you walk with purpose, stepping first on your heel, then pushing off to the next step with the ball of your foot, you've got the right idea. Remember that snake: always coiled, always ready. Keep your feet ready too.

When you march between movements or do punches with footwork, you increase your heart rate, your circulation, and your muscles' ability to respond. Footwork of any kind is also good for firming and strengthening your calves. Take the time and concentrate on these steps, especially if you're having trouble keeping in time or shifting comfortably between moves in combinations.

Marching

In Tae-Bo we march between moves to stay in rhythm. Remember: Everything we do in Tae-Bo is done on an eight count. You don't want to lose track of the count or fall off the beat of the music. That will only make it harder to get back into the movement again. Marching also keeps the body moving so your heart rate isn't constantly slowing down, then speeding up, then slowing down again. When you march, don't just shuffle your feet or walk as if you were on a treadmill. This isn't a rest. You've got to be ready to move into action after that eighth count.

1 Lift your feet from your knees, keeping your abs tight and your back straight.

2 Keep your feet softly flexed; don't point your toes.

3 And move those arms: With your elbows bent and your forearms up, make a controlled pumping motion with the fist opposite your stepping foot.

To make your marching more challenging:

▶ lift your knees as high as you can

To keep your marching from becoming too tiring:

▶ don't raise your knees as high, but be sure that your feet are coming up off the floor and you aren't just "walking in place"

Pivoting

Many Tae-Bo moves, sequences, and combinations demand quick changes in direction and weight distribution. To accomplish this safely, you must pivot easily and correctly. It's easier to pivot if you understand its purpose: to turn all the parts of your lower body so they move in the same direction and at the same time as your upper body.

It sounds simple enough, but pivoting correctly doesn't come easily to most people. For one thing, pivoting is a whole-body move. When we think of pivoting, we usually picture someone twisting at the hips or the waist or the knees. This is exactly the opposite of what a true pivot should be. Not only does twisting a single area limit your mobility, it makes you vulnerable to injury. The high rate of knee injury, even among professional athletes, in sports that demand a lot of pivoting movements—such as basketball, football, and skiing—gives you some idea of how important a good pivoting technique is.

Even if you think you know how to do it, take some time to check yourself. Instead of turning your whole body in the direction you're moving, you might turn only the top half of your body. This places unnecessary and potentially damaging stress on the knees, hips, and back. Just because you've exercised before doesn't mean you were taught the correct way to move. Chances are, if you were doing movements that called for twisting at the waist, you were probably told specifically to keep your feet planted on the floor, your hips facing forward, and not to pivot. When you do Tae-Bo, watch for old habits like these. They may be compromising your Workout and your safety.

Our bodies were not designed to work with one part pulling in the opposite direction of the other. When you fail to pivot, you hold your body back and limit the range and force of your movement. The results are a less powerful punch, a kick that's off-balance, and a lack of body confidence. To get the most out of Tae-Bo, you've got to face in the direction you're moving and put your whole body—from your head to your toes—behind it.

The Principles of Pivoting

- Always start in the correct position.

- Don't just think on your feet; think about them. Be aware of which part of your foot is the pivot point—the heel or the ball of your foot.

- Know in which direction the rest of your foot will be moving from that point. For example, punches always pivot from the ball of the foot and swing the heel in the direction opposite the move. So to execute a Right Cross—which travels from right to left—you pivot so your toes point left and your heels swing right. Some kicks, like the Side Kick and the Roundhouse, have the supporting leg and the lead, kicking leg pivoting in the same direction with the toes of both feet pointing opposite the direction of the kick.

- Think ahead: You will pivot in the direction you're going to move. The only exceptions are the Side Kick and the Roundhouse Kick, where you pivot your lower body in the direction opposite the one you're kicking in.

- Remember: Your feet are just the foundation. Turn everything else in the same direction simultaneously.

- Always look in the direction you're turning.

- If you feel like your feet are stuck to the floor, check your technique. If you're up on the balls of your feet and turning your whole body correctly, take a look at the floor and your feet. It's more difficult to pivot correctly on a thick carpet than a wooden floor or smoother, industrial-type floor covering. Also, check your shoes. Some have very deep, intricate tread designs that may catch on your floor. Try going barefoot or, if you're on carpet, wearing just your socks. Practicing this way, you may be able to improve your pivoting technique to the point where you can do it well on any surface.

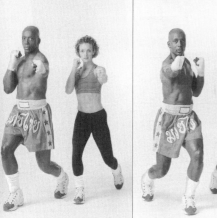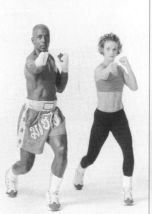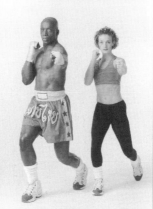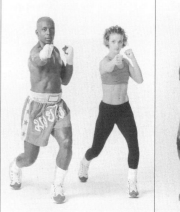

The Basic Pivot

1 Shift the weight on your pivoting foot from your heel to the ball of your foot. As you turn left, visualize a wire running from your right foot, through your right heel, hip, waist, rib cage, neck, and head, and turn your entire body *simultaneously.*

2 Always look in the direction you're turning.

3 When you pivot back to your starting position, turn every part of your body *simultaneously.*

Modified Pivot for Side Kick and Roundhouse Kick

In the martial arts, we refer to a position that sets up the body for another movement—such as a punch or a kick—as the "chamber." When you raise your leg into position for a kick, that's called chambering. Part of chambering for a Side Kick or a Roundhouse Kick involves pivoting with both feet so your heels face in the direction of the kick and your lead, or kicking, hip is aimed at your imaginary opponent. As you do this, remember:

- Pivot away from the kick instead of toward it.

- Do not turn your whole body in the direction of the pivot. As you pivot your lower body to chamber for the kick, your chest and abdomen remain facing frontward. If you turned your whole body to follow the pivot, you'd end up with your back facing your opponent, which would defeat the whole defensive purpose of these kicks.

- Pivot both feet simultaneously, concentrating your weight on the balls of your feet equally, then quickly shifting about 80 percent of your weight to the supporting, non-kicking leg.

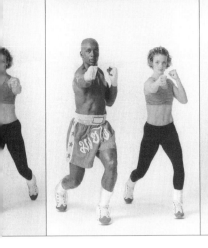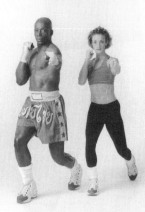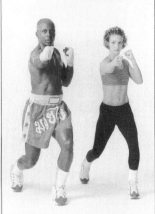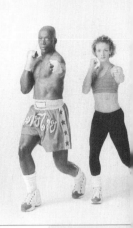

Bouncing Footwork

Bouncing footwork gives punches extra energy and bounce. It gives you a much better cardiovascular workout than just doing reps of punches alone. As you do your footwork, remember that you are not taking steps; this isn't like jogging or walking in place. You want to keep it smooth.

1 Starting from a Right Side Stance or a Left Side Stance, move in place on the balls of your feet.

2 Instead of moving up and down, get into a forward-and-backward motion that is controlled by your abs and your hips.

3 Concentrate on not surging forward and using your knees as brakes to stop your body weight. Don't lift your toes, and don't fall back down on your heels. Create the motion by shifting your weight easily and rapidly from foot to foot.

4 Keep your knees and your hips following the direction of your feet. They should be relaxed, never locked.

5 Keep your rib cage high, your abs tight, and your hips loose but level. They should be moving with your footwork, but not wiggling up and down with every step. If they are, you're probably not tightening up your abdominals enough, and you may be stressing your lower back. Also be aware of your hands, which should be punching or in a guard position, but not flailing around.

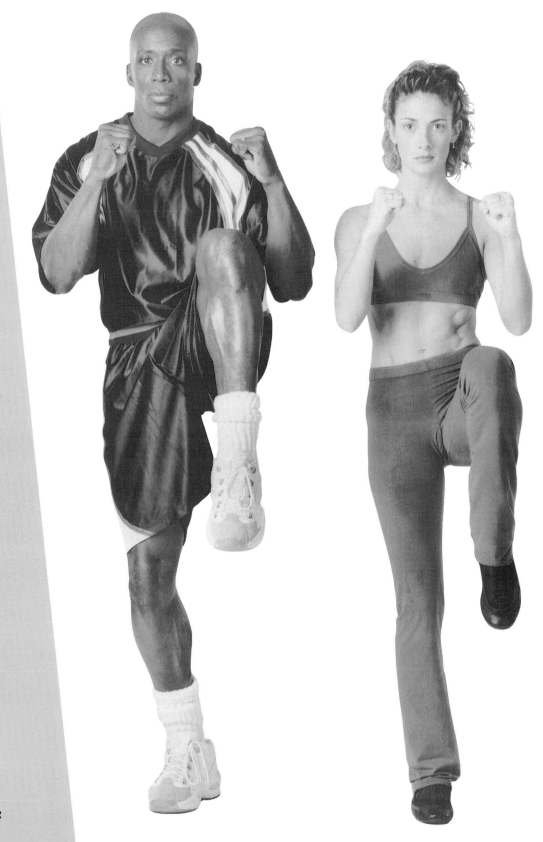

Knee Raises

In Tae-Bo, we use two Knee Raises: the Front Knee Raise and the Side Knee Raise. In the Front Knee Raise, the hip flexors raise the knee and chamber the leg in preparation for the Front Kick and a number of other exercises you'll find in the Advanced Tae-Bo Workouts. The Side Knee Raise uses the hip flexors and the abductors.

Knee Raises are an exercise in their own right, but they're also the key to the kick. Remember: The kick is an extension of a focused and carefully controlled Knee Raise.

The Principles of Knee Raises

- Keep in mind that you will be raising your back leg and that your supporting leg will be your front leg. This is the opposite of leg positioning for most other Tae-Bo moves.

- The weight of the leg you're raising should be concentrated in the ball of that foot, so you're ready to move. If you let that foot drop and concentrate your weight in your heel, it will be harder for you to raise your knee.

- Correct your balance by moving up and down slightly on your supporting leg. Don't move sideways or let your arms get out of guard position and away from your body.

- Always isolate the correct muscles and watch for signs that you're not. If you feel yourself leaning forward, hunching, or bending your torso forward to meet your leg and knee, stop. That's a sign you're not using your stomach muscles to stabilize your upper body as your hip flexors do the work.

- As with any Tae-Bo movement, be sure your leg follows the same path coming back that it did going out. That means you have to concentrate on telling your leg what to do. Remember: You have the brain; your leg doesn't.

- Understand that the correct stance and the correct Knee Raise are more than just preliminaries to the kick. The truth is, your kick can be only as good as the lift. Give them the time and attention they deserve.

- The height and direction of the actual kick are not determined by your foot but by how well you've positioned your body in your stance and your knee in the Knee Raise. The kick itself is really an isolated movement of your knee, your lower leg, and your foot.

Getting the Most Out of Knee Raises

Being able to execute a Side Knee Raise smoothly while maintaining your balance is important to giving your Tae-Bo Workout rhythm and flow, not to mention a great way to tighten up your abdominal muscles. The secret to executing quick repetitions of the Side Knee Raise and any related kick is keeping your stable leg slightly bent (but not so deeply that you can't see your toes) and allowing your other foot to lightly touch down—not land—on your toes or balls of your feet after each raise.

Your leg muscles are the largest and heaviest in your body, especially your glutes, your quads, and your calves. It takes more energy to move them, more concentration to keep those movements controlled, and more focus to keep your recovery clean every time. When these muscles start to tire, expect to feel it in a big way. It's not unusual to find yourself tiring more quickly during legwork than other parts of the Workout. But be aware. Don't drop your guard, not even for your own body. Expect your legs to feel tired. Expect to feel like cutting corners on your technique or your repetitions. Look out for the first time you might not be raising your knee as high as you could, or you let your leg drop back into standing position. When that happens, call on your mind and your spirit to refocus and get your legs back on track. Later, when you're doing kicks, you'll face the same challenges. Practice taking control now. (Although it might feel like your legs are doing most of the work, Knee Raises also work—and strengthen—your lower back, abs, hamstrings, and glutes.)

If you keep moving without focus, if you let the weight of those muscles fall, you're compromising your Workout. More important, you risk several different kinds of injury (lower back, ankles, knees, hips). Instead of using the correct muscles to bring your leg back into position, you end up straining other muscles and jarring your joints. Even if you have to slow down your pace, march a little, or shift to some arm movements for eight counts, don't give up. As soon as you can, get back into the Workout.

You can make your Knee Raises more challenging by:

▶ concentrating more on your abdominal muscles to stabilize your body as you raise your knee higher

▶ making your technique—especially on your recovery—as close to perfect as possible

▶ doing more reps

▶ not letting your foot touch down between raises

▶ combining all four of the points above in every single rep

You can help yourself do more reps of Knee Raises by:

▶ not raising your knee as high but maintaining good technique

▶ letting your foot touch down between raises

▶ pointing your toes when you raise your knee—this will make your leg feel lighter and work the front muscles of your leg

▶ flexing your foot when you raise your knee—this will work the muscles at the back of your leg, making your leg feel heavier, but also giving the muscles at the front of your leg a rest, so you can resume reps with your toes pointed and continue longer

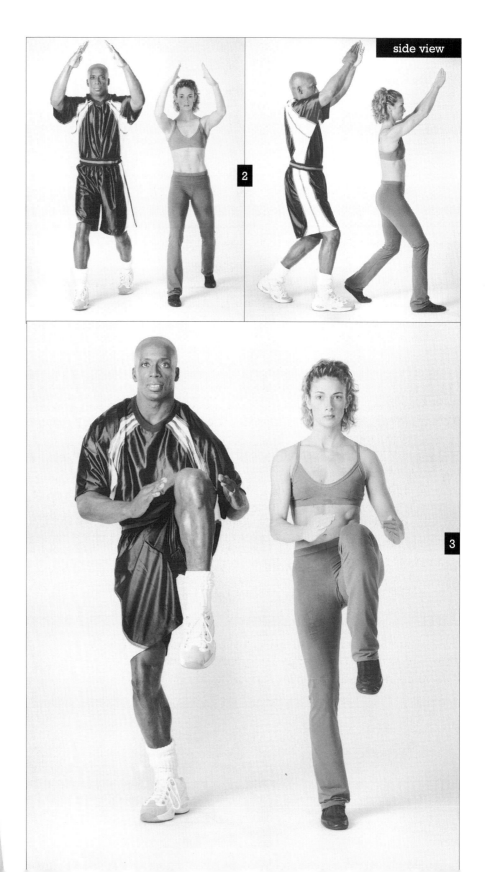

side view

2

3

116

THE FRONT KNEE RAISE

The Left Front Knee Raise

1 From a Forward Stance, step straight back with your left leg until your feet are about shoulder-distance apart and parallel. Your knees should be slightly bent, with your right leg forward, bearing about 80 percent of your weight. Your right foot is flat while your left foot is in position to move—bearing little weight and with the heel up.

2 Raise your arms from a forward guard position to reach above and slightly in front of your head, with your hands open, palms facing each other, elbows soft, and fingers pointing up.

3 Concentrating on stabilizing your upper body with your abdominal muscles, in one count, bring your arms down as you lift your left knee toward your belly button. Do not bend at the waist; keep your back straight, your rib cage high. Your left foot should be softly pointed and under your knee, not extended beyond it.

4 Return to start position, but be ready to move again. Don't fall back on a flat foot.

If this movement is part of a series of repetitions or a combination, remember to touch down lightly on your toes between raises. Try not to bounce or straighten the supporting leg completely.

The Right Front Knee Raise

1 From a Forward Stance, step straight back with your right leg until your feet are about shoulder-distance apart and parallel. Your knees should be slightly bent, with your left leg forward, bearing about 80 percent of your weight. Your left foot is flat while your right foot is in position to move—bearing little weight and with the heel up.

2 Raise your arms from a forward guard position to reach above and slightly in front of your head, with your hands open, palms facing each other, elbows soft, and fingers pointing up.

3 Concentrating on stabilizing your upper body with your abdominal muscles, in one count, bring your arms down as you lift your right knee toward your belly button. Do not bend at the waist; keep your back straight, your rib cage high. Your right foot should be softly pointed and under your knee, not extended beyond it.

4 Return to start position, but be ready to move again. Don't fall back on a flat foot.

If this movement is part of a series of repetitions or a combination, remember to touch down lightly on your toes between raises. Try not to bounce or straighten the supporting leg completely.

ALTERNATING FRONT KNEE RAISES

If you're alternating legs, make sure that you're shifting your weight from one stable leg to the other without bouncing or rocking. Check your hips. Make sure they're remaining fairly square and that you're not sinking down into the supporting leg or raising your hip as you raise your knee.

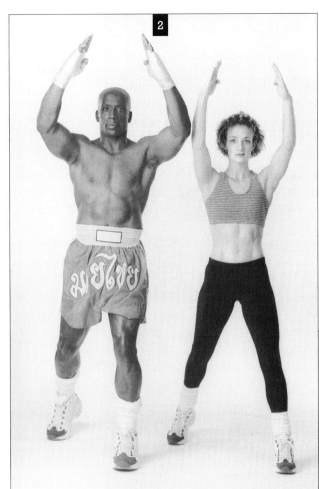

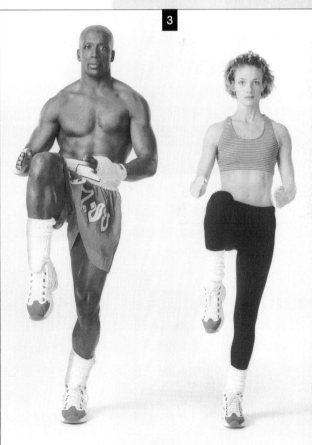

THE SIDE KNEE RAISE

The Side Knee Raise is the foundation for the Side Kick and the Roundhouse Kick. It's also part of some of the Floor Work and Combinations.

Like the Front Knee Raise, the Side Knee Raise also demands that your upper body be stabilized, and that works your abs. Then your hip flexors and abductors lift up your leg. Instead of raising your knee toward your belly button, imagine that you're pulling your entire upper leg up toward your opposite shoulder from the side.

Another point on positioning: Like the Front Knee Raise, you execute the Side Knee Raise with your back leg, not your leading leg. Notice that you begin a Left Side Knee Raise from a Right Side Stance and a Right Side Knee Raise from a Left Side Stance.

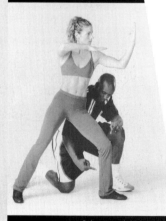

correct knee and
back foot position

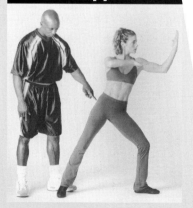

correct hip position

The Left Side Knee Raise

1 Start in the Forward Stance, then move into a Right Side Stance by taking a step straight back with your left leg. Your feet will be facing forward, about shoulder-distance apart and parallel—though not side by side. Your arms should be extended upward, a few inches in front of you and slightly to the right.

2 With about 80 percent of your weight on your slightly bent, supporting right leg, and the rest on the ball—not the heel—of your left foot, find your balance. Be sure your right knee does not extend beyond your right toes.

3 Raise your left leg so your knee is being drawn up diagonally across your body and toward your right shoulder. Keep your left foot softly flexed. Now really contract your abs for stability, bring your arms down, and exhale as you pull your leg up.

4 Lower your left leg—following the same path back—and return to start position.

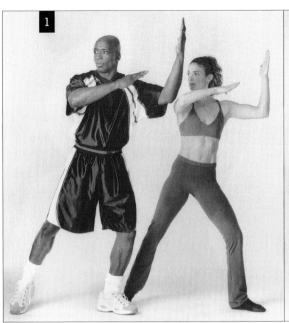

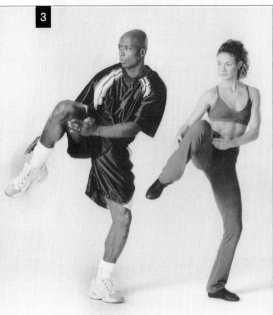

The Right Side Knee Raise

1 Start in the Forward Stance, then move into a Left Side Stance by taking a step straight back with your right leg. Your feet will be facing forward, about shoulder-distance apart and parallel—though not side by side. Your arms should be extended upward, a few inches in front of you and slightly to the left.

2 With about 80 percent of your weight on your slightly bent, supporting left leg, and the rest on the ball—not the heel—of your right foot, find your balance. Be sure your left knee does not extend beyond your left toes.

3 Raise your right leg so your knee is being drawn up diagonally across your body and toward your left shoulder. Keep your right foot softly flexed. Now really contract your abs for stability, bring your arms down, and exhale as you pull your leg up.

4 Lower your right leg—following the same path back—and return to start position.

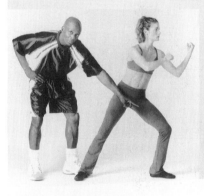

What's Wrong with This Picture?

The Side Knee Raise

X *Shellie's knee of her front, supporting leg is extending beyond her toes. This is going to compromise her balance and may injure her knee.*

X *Shellie is leaning forward and too far over to the side. Her hip has sunk down, which will make it harder for her to pick up her knee.*

X *Shellie's guard is sloppy–it's too far away from her body to protect her.*

121

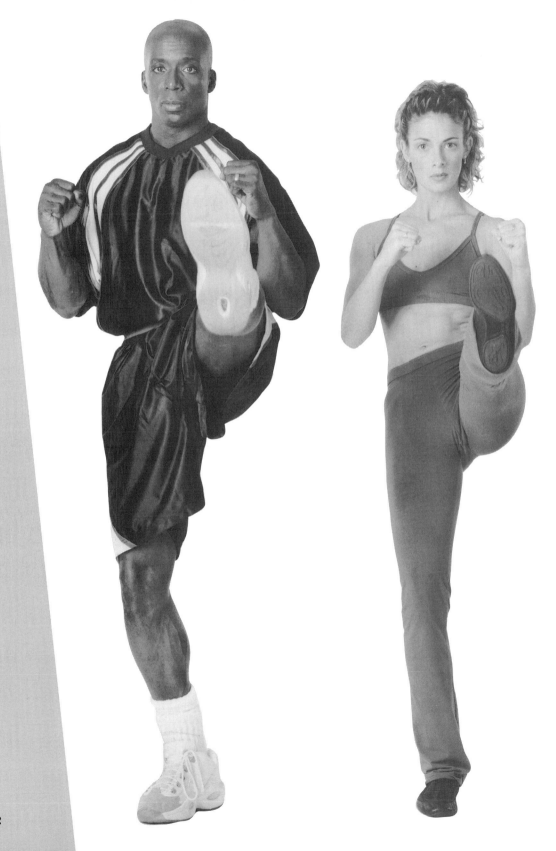

the Kicks

The kicks are probably the most dramatic moves in Tae-Bo. They're harder in some ways and more tiring than anything else we do. But they also make you stronger, because they work the muscles that shape your butt, your thighs, your legs, and your abs.

Throughout this section, I explain how these kicks are used in martial arts, to show the purpose of different positions. It also helps you visualize the angle and the direction of your body and your kick.

The Principles of Kicks

Each kick in Tae-Bo has its own technique. As you learn to do each, always keep these points in mind. Not only will they help you work more comfortably and more safely, they'll help you achieve the best kick you can.

- Always look in the direction that you're kicking and have a focus point.
- Exhale at the point of impact; inhale on the chambering moves and recovery.
- Never fully extend your kicking leg. The point of impact of your kick should be two to three inches short of full extension.
- Always keep your supporting leg bent, but not so deeply that you can't see your toes. Never lock your knees.
- Use your hip flexors and, for the Side Kick, the abductors to raise your knee and your leg. Never kick straight from the hip or swing your leg from your hip.
- Maintain your balance by keeping your arms close to your body. If you still feel off balance, compensate by moving up or down slightly (no more than a couple of inches) on your bent supporting leg, not from side to side.
- As you're kicking, always use your abs to keep your chest and abdomen upright and stable. Remember that pillar: That's your strength.
- Focus on the position of your foot. Some people concentrate so much on the abs, the legs, the arms, and everything else they're working, they just let their kicking foot flop. Correct foot position is essential. For the Side Kick, your foot should be flexed, so the point of contact is the side of the foot, while for the Roundhouse Kick, your foot should be pointed, so the point of contact is the top of the foot. For the Front Kick, you can flex your foot to work muscles at the back of the leg, or point it to work muscles in the front.
- If you have trouble pointing your toes, try working out barefoot. Sometimes your shoe can limit your foot's range of motion.

◘ As with any Tae-Bo movement, be sure your leg follows the same path coming back that it did going out. That means you have to concentrate on telling your leg what to do. I promise you, that will get harder to do as your muscles begin to tire. But always tell yourself who's the boss: It's you, not your leg.

◘ Kick to where you feel most comfortable. Remember: A lower kick with good technique is better than a higher kick with sloppy technique. You can kick lower. That's okay. But always keep working toward that higher kick, even if the difference is only an inch or two. It's always better to work with a goal in mind.

Now, there are people who can kick as high as their shoulder, and one day, you may be able to do that too. But you don't need to do that now, or ever. Remember: A high kick doesn't work your muscles any more than a lower kick. And a high kick is not necessarily a correct kick. Focus on achieving the best possible technique at whatever height you can reach comfortably. Again, concentrate on that knee. It's important, because wherever your knee points once your leg is raised, that will be the direction of your kick.

To make your kicks more challenging:

▶ kick a little bit higher than you think you can

▶ kick to a different height with each set, or vary the heights from kick to kick (for example, to the knee, to the hip, to the head)

▶ concentrate on keeping your upper body, your arms, and your supporting leg in perfect position

▶ don't let your kicking foot come down completely to the floor between reps

▶ do more reps on each side

To make it possible for you to do more reps:

▶ on Front Kicks, alternate between flexing and pointing your foot between sets

▶ kick lower, but continue to use good technique

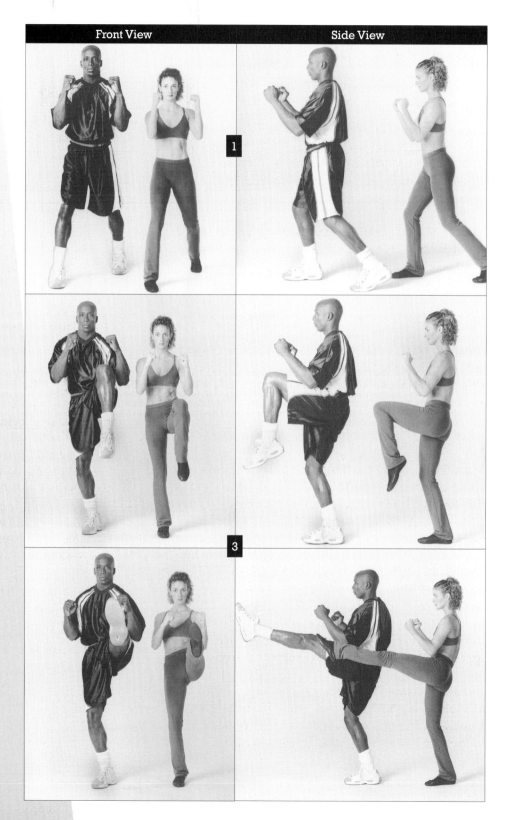

THE FRONT KICK

The Left Front Kick

1 Start in a Forward Stance, then move into a Right Side Stance by taking a step straight back with your left leg. Your feet will be facing forward, about shoulder-distance apart and parallel—though not side by side. Your hands should be up in guard position.

2 With about 80 percent of your weight on your slightly bent, supporting right leg, and the rest on the ball—not the heel—of your left foot, find your balance.

3 With your left foot pointed, do a Front Knee Raise, then kick straight out to two to three inches short of full extension.

4 Immediately retract your foot, bringing it back down to the Front Knee Raise position *before* letting it touch down in the start position. Remember: Your foot, knee, and leg should travel the same route on recovery they took in execution.

The Right Front Kick

1 Start in a Forward Stance, then move into a Left Side Stance by taking a step straight back with your right leg. Your feet will be facing forward, about shoulder-distance apart and parallel—though not side by side. Your hands should be up in guard position.

2 With about 80 percent of your weight on your slightly bent, supporting left leg, and the rest on the ball—not the heel—of your right foot, find your balance.

3 With your right foot pointed, do a Front Knee Raise, then kick straight out to two to three inches short of full extension.

4 Immediately retract your foot, bringing it back down to the Front Knee Raise position *before* letting it touch down in the start position. Remember: Your foot, knee, and leg should travel the same route on recovery they took in execution.

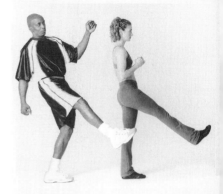

What's Wrong with This Picture?

The Front Kick

X *I'm swinging my leg from my hip instead of kicking from a raised knee. Not only is there no power behind this swinging kick, I'm off-balance, losing control, and risking injury to my knee and my hip.*

X *I'm letting my kicking leg fall back down into the start position instead of taking it first to the Front Knee Raise and then down to the start position from there. This sloppy technique isn't giving me the benefits of the Workout, and I'm risking injury.*

X *At the point of impact, Shellie's leg is totally extended and her knee is locked.*

THE FRONT KICK, SITTING IN A CHAIR

You can still work your legs, your back, and your abs by doing a Front Kick from a chair. The key to getting results is to really focus on working the correct muscles and controlling every stage of the move.

1 Sit in a firm chair that has a straight back. Try to sit up as straight as you can. The straighter your back, the more fully you'll be able to work your abs. You can sit with your back against the chair back as long as you're not leaning against it.

2 Begin with your feet flat on the ground in front of you. Raise one leg toward your stomach as high as you comfortably can.

3 Execute the kick, stopping two to three inches short of full extension.

4 Recover your leg carefully. Don't let your leg drop. Repeat for 8 reps, then switch sides.

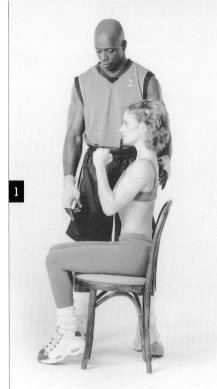

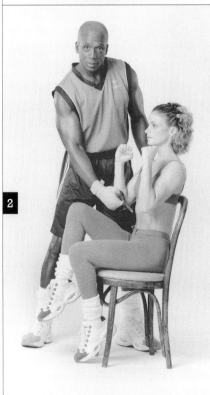

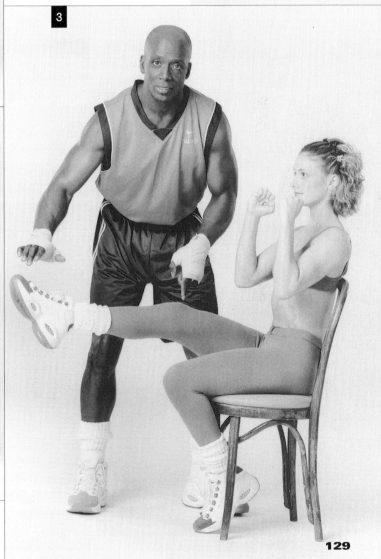

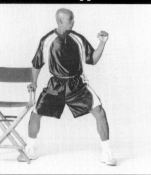

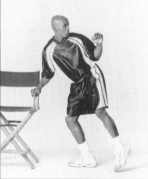

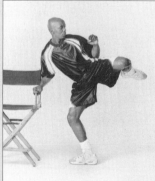

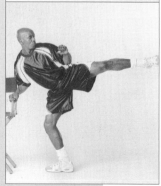

Using Support for Balance

Learning to find and keep your balance takes time, practice, and patience. If you don't feel confident while doing these moves, you can work on your technique while your balance improves. This isn't cheating, because it's making it possible for you to do Tae-Bo. And Tae-Bo—even when you're doing moves with extra support—develops balance. There's nothing wrong with using a chair for as long as you feel you need to. I'm confident, though, that after a while, you'll find yourself relying on the chair less and less. During each Workout, test yourself. If you're resting your entire hand on the chair back, try using your fingers, then try two fingers, then one, then none.

Even though you're using something for support, the way you execute the kick will be exactly the same as if you were standing without support.

If you use a chair, a bar, or a countertop for support, keep this in mind:

◻ Be sure whatever you're using for support is stable and not likely to shift or collapse. (For example, do not use a folding chair.)

◻ Stand the correct distance away. You should be able to stand straight and use your hand for support without reaching (which means you're too far away) or bending (which means you're too close).

◻ Remember that you're using the chair only for balance. If you find yourself leaning on it or placing your weight against it to help you raise your knee higher, for example, stop. True Tae-Bo is perfecting whatever movement you can execute comfortably, even if you can't yet raise your leg to kick very high. If you're using the support for more than balance, you may be picking up bad habits that you'll have to unlearn to do the Workout.

◻ Test yourself every day, on every movement. You'll be surprised at how quickly your balance can increase.

◻ Use the support selectively, only when you really need it. Everyone comes to Tae-Bo with different abilities. Just because you have trouble finding your balance in one position doesn't mean you can't find it in others. Be aware of your body. You may discover you don't need the support for the Knee Raise, but still could use a little extra help for the kick.

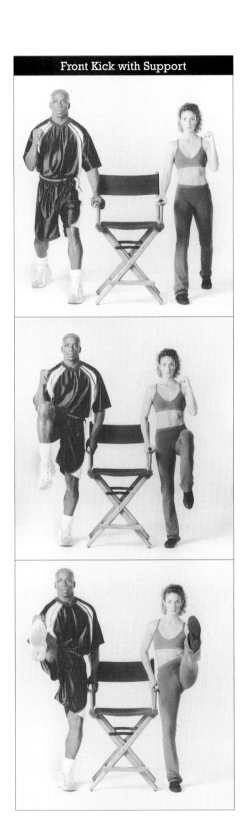

Front Kick with Support

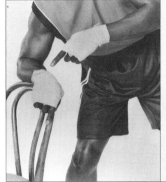

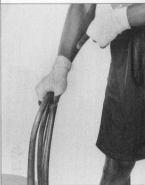

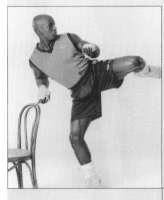

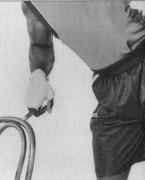

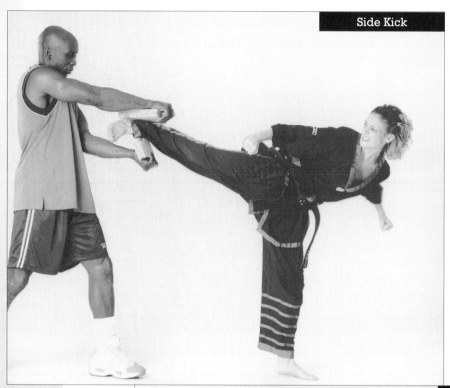

Side Kick

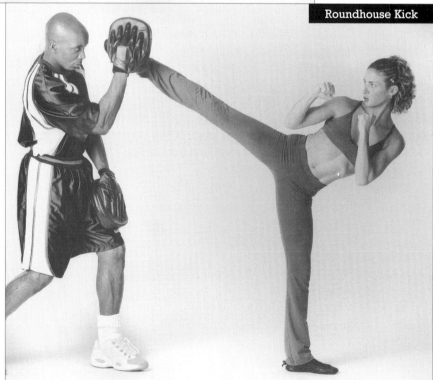

Roundhouse Kick

The Side Kick and the Roundhouse Kick: What Makes the Difference?

Students who are new to Tae-Bo sometimes have trouble distinguishing a Side Kick from a Roundhouse Kick. That's understandable, because the two kicks have a lot in common and their differences may not be obvious from videos or pictures. You may find it easier to focus on your kicks if you understand these differences.

In the martial arts, the Side Kick and the Roundhouse Kick serve two different purposes. The Side Kick is a very powerful kick, aimed at an opponent coming directly toward your kicking foot. Since the goal is to kick your opponent with full force, you focus on using muscles in your butt and your hips to drive a hard flexed foot straight out (but a few inches short of full extension), in a jabbing motion that makes the heel of your foot the point of contact. If you think of the Side Kick as the Jab of kicks, then the Roundhouse Kick is more like a backhand slap. It's used to catch an oncoming opponent on his side. Instead of thrusting your lower leg out Side Kick style, you want to visualize whipping your lower leg from the knee down, so that the top of your foot (with your toes pointed) snaps your opponent from the side.

In these photos of Shellie demonstrating these kicks (and, no, I don't expect you to kick that high—yet), you can see the difference clearly. The Side Kick is the kick she uses to break a board. The Roundhouse Kick is the kick she'd use to knock that board out of my hand from its side.

Whichever kick you're doing, remember to position your body in a way that offers your imaginary opponent the smallest amount of exposed body space. That means you face in the direction of the kicks but your upper body—shoulders, chest, abdomen—all remain facing frontward. It's also important to keep your back from turning or curving away from the kick. This not only makes you vulnerable to your invisible opponent, but it will throw off your kick.

Also, remember to always start your kick from the correct position. For both the Side Kick and the Roundhouse Kick, that means pivoting both feet in the direction opposite the kick and positioning your hip so that it points upward and in line with the kick. At the same time, you must be sure that your upper body remains open and facing forward. In other words, don't let your upper body twist toward the kick. Instead, your upper body should be leaning slightly in the direction opposite the kick, over your supporting leg. If you think in terms of self-defense, these fine points of positioning will make more sense to you and be easier to remember. What you're trying to do is expose the smallest amount of body area to your opponent. You don't hunch or twist away from the kick, because you won't be able to see your opponent.

THE SIDE KICK

The secret to executing solid, quick kicks is learning the technique so well that it becomes second nature to you. We break these kicks down because there are many important details to keep in mind as you learn, but don't let them overwhelm you. As your technique improves, you'll find yourself moving into the correct position almost automatically. In the meantime, take it as easily as you need to until you're ready to bring your kick up to speed.

The Left Side Kick

1. Start from a Horse Stance, then move into a Left Horse Stance by turning only your head so you're facing left, the direction of your kick. The rest of your body should be facing forward.

2. With your right foot, take a decisive step sideways, so your feet are two to six inches apart. Immediately pivot both feet so as you bring your right foot down, both feet are turned right and both heels are fully facing left. Shift about 80 percent of your weight to your slightly bent, supporting right leg. The small remainder of the weight on your left foot should be concentrated in the ball of your foot, so you're ready to move.

3. Here's what makes this a Side Kick: In one movement, lift your left heel and knee as high as you comfortably can. However high that is, it's important that your left heel and knee be at the same level. You may find your upper body leaning to your right to compensate for balance. As you do, be sure you are not turning your left shoulder to the right, turning at the waist to the right, or hunching. Your shoulders and chest should be facing frontward and open.

4. Quickly kick out about two to three inches short of full extension. Your left foot should be flexed. This kick should be lightning quick, with no time between the impact and recovery. Strive to kick out without moving your shoulders, rising on your supporting leg, or letting your weight drop on the supporting leg.

5. Retract your foot and be sure you reach the full Knee Raise before touching down with your left foot. Remember: Bring your leg back in following the same path it went out on, using the exact but reversed order of positions.

6. Lower your left leg so your feet are together. Shift your weight so it's equally distributed, and step right with your right foot back into the starting Horse Stance.

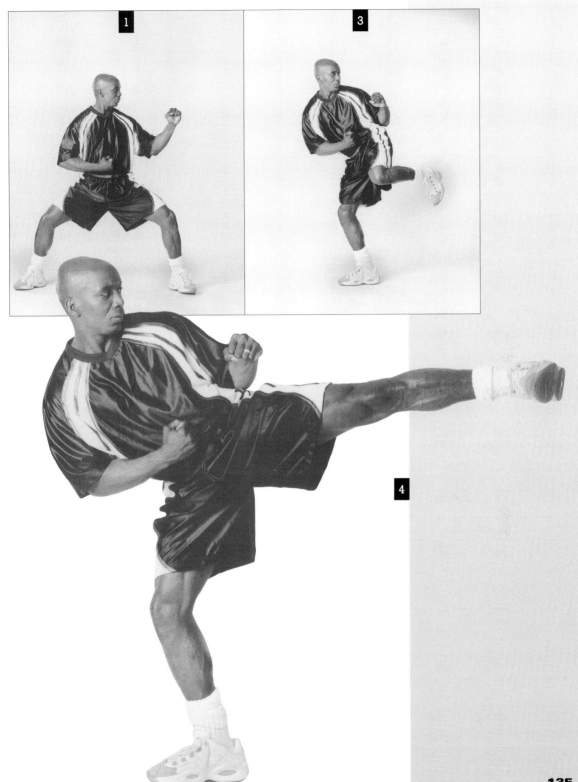

The Right Side Kick

1 Start from a Horse Stance, then move into a Right Horse Stance by turning only your head so you're facing right, the direction of your kick. The rest of your body should be facing forward.

2 With your left foot, take a decisive step sideways, so your feet are only two to six inches apart. Immediately pivot both feet so as you bring your left foot down, both feet are turned left and both heels are fully facing right. Shift about 80 percent of your weight to your slightly bent, supporting left leg. The small remainder of the weight on your right foot should be concentrated in the ball of your foot, so you're ready to move.

3 Here's what makes this a Side Kick: In one movement, lift your right heel and knee as high as you comfortably can. However high that is, it's important that your right heel and knee be at the same level. You may find your upper body leaning to your left to compensate for balance. As you do, be sure you are not turning your right shoulder to the left, turning at the waist to the left, or hunching. Your shoulders and chest should be facing frontward and open.

4 Quickly kick out about two to three inches short of full extension. Your right foot should be flexed. This kick should be lightning quick, with no time between the impact and recovery. Strive to kick out without moving your shoulders, rising on your supporting leg, or letting your weight drop on the supporting leg.

5 Retract your foot and be sure you reach the full Knee Raise before touching down with your right foot. Remember: Bring your leg back in following the same path it went out on, using the exact but reversed order of positions.

6 Lower your right leg so your feet are together. Shift your weight so it's equally distributed, and step left with your left foot back into the starting Horse Stance.

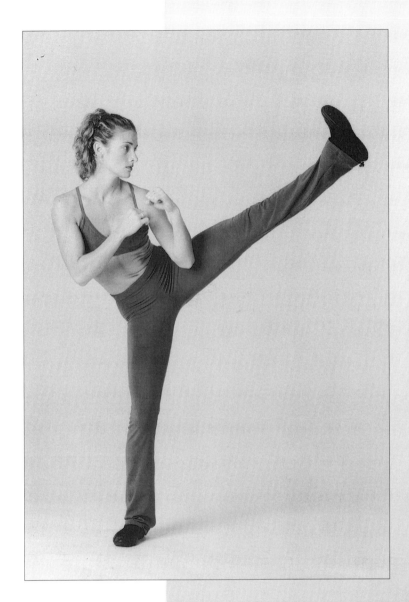

What's Wrong with This Picture?

The Side Kick

- ☒ Shellie's right supporting leg is totally straight, and her left kicking leg is completely extended.

- ☒ Shellie's guard is too loose. By holding her arms down in front of her, she's more likely to bend at the waist and direct her kick to the front of her body instead of the side.

- ☒ Shellie isn't using her upper body to help power her kick. She's holding her upper body far too straight, and that's making it harder for her to push the kick out.

- ☒ Instead of keeping her upper body facing forward, she's turning her left shoulder away from her kick and twisting her body. This will make it more difficult for her to recover her kick.

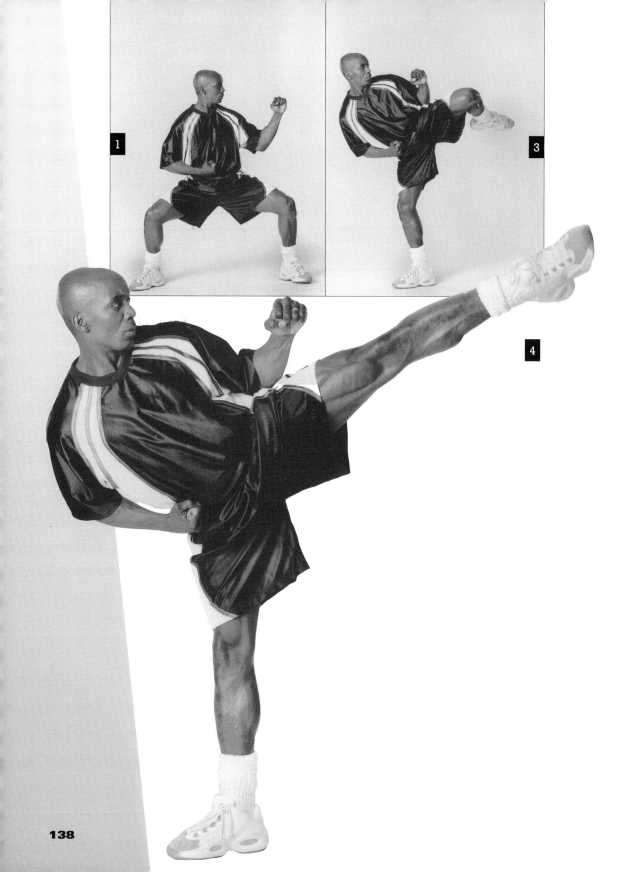

THE ROUNDHOUSE KICK

The Left Roundhouse Kick

1 Start from a Horse Stance, then move into a Left Horse Stance by turning only your head so you're facing left, the direction of your kick. The rest of your body should be facing forward.

2 With your right foot, take a decisive step sideways, so your feet are only a few inches apart. Immediately pivot both feet so as you bring your right foot down, both feet are turned right and both heels are fully facing left. Shift about 80 percent of your weight to your slightly bent, supporting right leg. The small remainder of the weight on your left foot should be concentrated in the ball of your foot, so you're ready to move.

3 Here's what makes this a Roundhouse Kick: In one movement, lift your left heel and knee so they are at the same level and parallel to the floor. Go as high as you comfortably can. However high that is, it's important that the heel and knee be at the same level. You may find your upper body leaning to your right to compensate for balance. As you do, be sure you are not turning your left shoulder to the right, turning at the waist to the right, or hunching. Your shoulders and chest should be facing frontward and open.

4 With your kicking foot in a hard point, quickly kick in a whiplike motion from your knee, stopping two to three inches short of full extension. This kick should be lightning quick, with just an instant between the impact and recovery. Strive to kick out without moving your shoulders, rising on your supporting leg, or letting your weight drop on the supporting leg.

5 Retract your foot so your lifted knee is bent and your heel is behind your lifted thigh. Be sure you reach the full Knee Raise before touching down with your left foot. Remember: Bring your leg back in following the same path it went out on, using the exact but reversed order of positions.

6 Lower your left leg so that your feet are together. Shift your weight so that it's equally distributed, and step right with your right foot back into the starting Horse Stance.

7 When you're doing a series of repetitions, be sure to tap down with the left foot as you move from the kick stance to the Left Horse Stance start position.

This is how you should be positioned after you take that step, before you chamber your kicking leg, for the Roundhouse Kick. Notice that both of Shellie's heels are turned in the direction of the kick and both feet are pointed in the opposite direction. Her knees are both slightly bent. At the same time, notice that her upper body is facing forward, so only her right side is exposed to her imaginary opponent. She is not turning away from the kick and exposing her back, even though her feet are pointed in that direction.

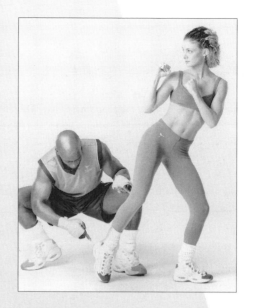

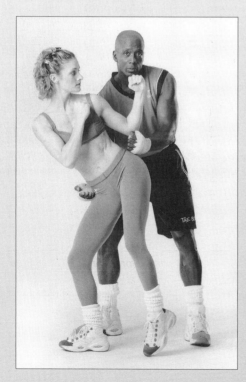

Pay special attention to this photograph, because it can take focus to chamber your kicking leg (in this picture, Shellie will be doing a Left Roundhouse Kick) without bending a little at the waist and turning your upper body in the opposite direction. The key to maintaining the correct technique throughout this kick is positioning your hip correctly before you raise your leg to kick. Notice that Shellie is raising her left hip up barely a few inches—just enough to raise her left heel up off the floor. Most important, though, she isn't just lifting her hip up, but actually pointing it at the imaginary target of her kick. At this point, 80 percent of her weight has been shifted to her supporting leg in preparation for the kick.

The Right Roundhouse Kick

1 Start from a Horse Stance, then move into a Right Horse Stance by turning only your head so you're facing right, the direction of your kick. The rest of your body should be facing forward.

2 With your left foot, take a decisive step sideways, so your feet are only a few inches apart. Immediately pivot both feet so as you bring your left foot down, both feet are turned left and both heels are fully facing right. Shift about 80 percent of your weight to your slightly bent, supporting left leg. The small remainder of the weight on your right foot should be concentrated in the ball of your foot, so you're ready to move.

3 Here's what makes this a Roundhouse Kick: In one movement, lift your right heel and knee so they are at the same level and parallel to the floor. Go as high as you comfortably can. However high that is, it's important that the heel and knee be at the same level. You may find your upper body leaning to your left to compensate for balance. As you do, be sure you are not turning your right shoulder to the left, turning at the waist to the left, or hunching. Your shoulders and chest should be facing frontward and open.

4 With your kicking foot in a hard point, quickly kick in a whip-like motion from your knee, stopping two to three inches short of full extension. This kick should be lightning quick, with just an instant between the impact and recovery. Strive to kick out without moving your shoulders, rising on your supporting leg, or letting your weight drop on the supporting leg.

5 Retract your foot so your lifted knee is bent and your heel is behind your lifted thigh. Be sure you reach the full Knee Raise before touching down with your right foot. Remember: Bring your leg back in following the same path it went out on, using the exact but reversed order of positions.

6 Lower your right leg so that your feet are together. Shift your weight so that it's equally distributed, and step left with your left foot back into the starting Horse Stance.

7 When you're doing a series of repetitions, be sure to tap down with the right foot as you move from the kick stance to the Right Horse Stance start position.

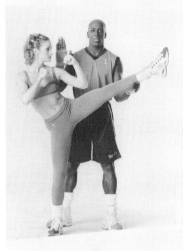

What's Wrong with This Picture?

The Roundhouse Kick

x *Shellie's hip and kicking foot are in the wrong position.*

x *Shellie's supporting leg is straight and her knee is locked instead of being slightly bent.*

x *Shellie's kicking leg hasn't been positioned properly, so she's just swung her leg up straight.*

x *Shellie isn't leaning away from her kick with her upper body.*

x *This kick can't have any force, and Shellie's balance is weak.*

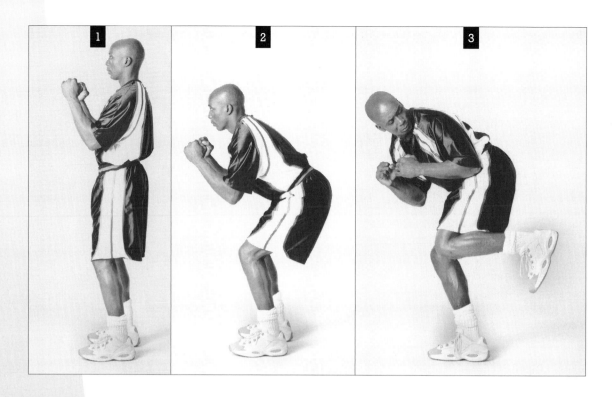

THE BACK KICK

The Back Kick is the most powerful kick in martial arts, because you put your largest, strongest muscle—the gluteus maximus—behind it. All that power also makes the Back Kick the easiest to do incorrectly. Many beginners have trouble with this one because it's not a common, natural motion and because they can't see the kick as clearly as they can see others.

In the instructions, you'll see that it's important to glance over your shoulder in the direction of the kick. However, some people find that even turning their heads slightly causes them to lose balance. If you find this happening, and you're working out in a room where you don't have to worry about kicking anyone or anything, try not looking to your side or behind you. Focus straight ahead and concentrate on improving your balance for this kick. Keep in mind that even though this makes the kick easier for you, it's also the beginning of a habit you'll want to break as soon as you can. As it becomes easier for you, start glancing over your shoulder with your peripheral vision. Simply turning your head slightly for an instant will give you enough of a view that you'll be safe.

No matter what condition you're in now, take this kick slow and easy. It's easy to execute if you start off in the right stance and don't overextend your leg on the kick. Aim for technique first, even if that means taking it at half-time when you can double-time everything else. As always, don't worry about how high you're kicking. Control is more important.

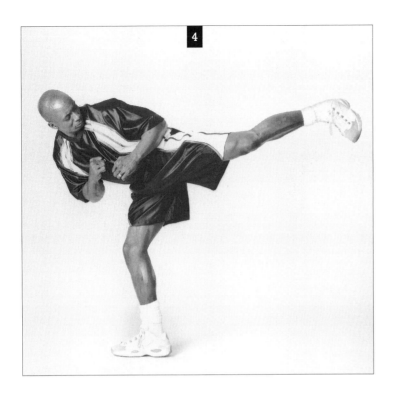

The Left Back Kick

1 Start in a Forward Stance, with your feet facing forward and parallel to each other, about shoulder-width apart. Your knees should be slightly bent, and your hands should be up in your guard. Start with your weight distributed equally between both legs.

2 Lower your weight by squatting a little deeper. Keep your back straight by bending forward at your hips—not your waist. Keep your back straight; don't round it or hunch it. Remember to keep your guard up too. That will help you keep your balance.

3 Shifting about 80 percent of your weight onto your supporting right leg, focus on raising your left leg, leading with your left heel. Then kick straight out behind you with a hard, flexed foot, and stop two to three inches short of full extension.

4 As you kick back, turn your head slightly to the left and glance over your left shoulder in the direction of the kick, using only your peripheral vision. Remember: Wherever your eyes look, your body tends to turn. If you turn your head all the way, you'll lose your balance.

5 Pull your left, kicking leg back in and return to start position. Be sure your kicking leg follows the exact path back that it took on its way out.

6 If you're going to be doing more reps of the Left Back Kick, bring your left foot down on the ball.

143

The Right Back Kick

1 Start in a Forward Stance, with your feet facing forward and parallel to each other, about shoulder-width apart. Your knees should be slightly bent, and your hands should be up in your guard. Start with your weight distributed equally between both legs.

2 Lower your weight by squatting a little deeper. Keep your back straight by bending forward at your hips—not your waist. Keep your back straight; don't round it or hunch it. Remember to keep your guard up too. That will help you keep your balance.

3 Shifting about 80 percent of your weight onto your supporting left leg, focus on raising your right leg, leading with your right heel. Then kick straight out behind you with a hard, flexed foot, and stop two to three inches short of full extension.

4 As you kick back, turn your head slightly to the right and glance over your right shoulder in the direction of the kick, using only your peripheral vision. Remember: Wherever your eyes look, your body tends to turn. If you turn your head all the way, you'll lose your balance.

5 Pull your right, kicking leg back in and return to start position. Be sure your kicking leg follows the exact path back that it took on its way out.

6 If you're going to be doing more reps of the Right Back Kick, bring your right foot down on the ball.

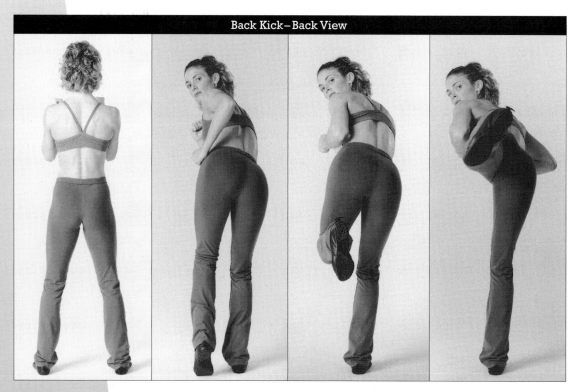

Back Kick–Back View

144

Alternating Back Kicks

When you alternate sides, the kick stays exactly the same. What does change is your ability to shift weight from leg to leg and keep your upper body stable and your hips level. If you're doing alternating Back Kicks, starting with a Left Back Kick, and the next kick will be with your right leg, bring your left foot down on your heel. This way you can more easily shift your weight so that your left leg becomes your supporting leg.

If you find it difficult to alternate Back Kicks without feeling like you're jerking when you kick and losing some of your balance during the transition from one side to the other, slow it down.

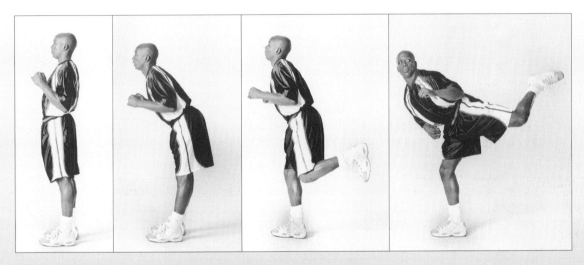

What's Wrong with This Picture?

The Back Kick

- ☒ My starting position is totally wrong. My knees are locked when they should be slightly bent.

- ☒ Even though my arms are in what looks like a guard position, it's weak and sloppy. It's a position without a purpose. My hands are down too low, and my arms aren't tight.

- ☒ Moving my weight down to position for the kick, my guard isn't up in the appropriate position.

- ☒ My knees are locked when they should be slightly bent.

- ☒ I'm extending my neck up and away from my body. It should be in a more natural position, with my chin down and looking straight ahead.

- ☒ I'm not glancing over my shoulder to see where I'm kicking.

- ☒ Instead of keeping my back straight as I bend forward from the hip, I'm bending at the waist, rounding my upper back, and throwing my leg out behind me.

- ☒ My recovery is weak; my foot's about to drop to the floor instead of coming back to the starting position in a smooth, controlled movement.

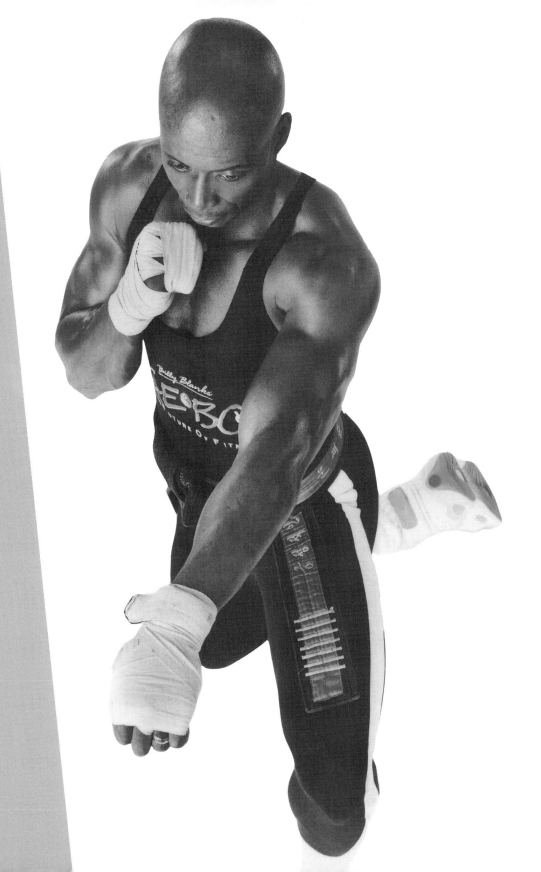

Tae-Bo's upper-body work revolves around four basic punches: the Jab, the Hook, the Uppercut, and the Cross. In fighting, each serves a different purpose, and understanding how they're applied can help you improve your technique, even though the only opponent you'll ever face in Tae-Bo will be an imaginary one. The Jab puts distance between you and an opponent in front of you. The Hook travels a half-circle away from your body and comes at an opponent from the side, the same way a Roundhouse Kick does. The Uppercut delivers a powerful blow at close range. And the Cross is the knockout punch that, in fighting, usually follows a Jab.

Like many people, you may find that punching feels weird to you. Unless you've trained to fight before or have been in situations where you've had to defend yourself, you probably haven't thrown more than a hundred punches in your life (in Tae-Bo, you'll be doing about four hundred each Workout). You are not alone. Very few women were taught even the bare basics of punching. Even among men today, the common knowledge about self-defense that once was handed down from fathers and older brothers to boys is a lost art. When you think about the world we live in, I find this hard to understand. How much safer would you feel if you knew how to punch? How much better would you feel if you knew your wife or husband, your daughter or your son, knew how to defend themselves?

Punches are fun to do. They feel great, and they tone just about everything: your abs, lats, waist, shoulders, biceps, and triceps. They'll help tighten up those flabby upper arms and melt away those love handles. When done correctly after a good Warm-up, punches also help reduce neck and upper-back tension. And a solid series of punches with lots of reps will get your heart pumping.

What you do with your fist and your arm is only a small part of a punch. It might help you to think of your punching arm as an arrow and the rest of your body as the bow. To deliver a focused, powerful punch, you have to put your whole body behind it. That means your shoulders, your back, your abdominals, your hips, your legs, and your feet turn in to the punch, creating an explosive motion that sends that punch out and snaps it right back with the same degree of force. It's important to always remember that a punch doesn't end when it makes contact with its target (even if that's just an imaginary spot in the air). A punch is never complete until you recover your fist and return to your starting stance. That's why focus and control are so important. Without them, a punch is nothing more than a fancy arm lift. You also run the risk of possible injury to your elbow, shoulder, knees, and back. Finally, students who don't follow through on the full punch fall out of time and struggle to get back into the count.

As you practice your punches, remember that you always want to feel the force at every step. Even as you stand in your starting position—*always* with your guard up—you should feel strong, alert, and ready for anything.

Study and practice the correct technique, but don't overthink it. Punches, like all the other Tae-Bo movements, are based on natural, everyday movements. I tell students who are learning to punch to visualize reaching out to give something to someone else, because the hand leads the arm out and back. A punch is no different, and keeping this in mind will prevent you from lifting your elbow when you punch.

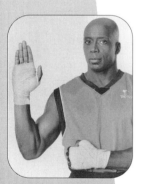 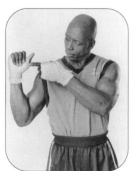 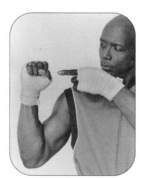 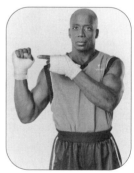

The Principles of Punching

The correct form begins with making the correct fist. With your palm open, roll your fingers inward to form a fist. Bend your thumb and press it firmly against the middle phalanges (those three sections of each finger) of your index and middle fingers. Be careful not to overextend your thumb to reach across all four fingers. This will make you bend your wrist upward and make it difficult to direct your arm.

- Your fist should be strong, tight, and ready to move. But it shouldn't be so tense that you feel the tension in your wrists and arms. Some people mistake tense muscles for strong muscles. In fact, the more comfortably relaxed you can be, the harder you'll probably punch, because you'll be moving and breathing correctly.

- Even though you're punching only air, follow the same form and punch with the same force you'd use against a physical target, such as a bag or an opponent. This will improve your technique and prevent injury. Use your entire body to drive the punch while focusing on the small area of your fist that will make contact at the moment of impact: the large, or first, knuckles of your index and middle fingers.

- Be aware of the position of your punching wrist and fist in relation to your arm. In a Jab, Hook, or Cross, your elbow, wrist, and fist should all form a single, unbroken line in perfect alignment. Anything else—say, for example, your fist is higher or lower than your wrist, or your wrist is higher or lower than your elbow—will be more difficult to control and may increase your chance of injury.

- No matter what punch you're doing, never fully extend your arm or lock your elbow. If you have trouble controlling your arm, try punching more slowly and deliberately until you instinctively know where to start pulling your punch back. Focus on finding that otherwise invisible, imaginary point in space that will be your target.

- If you're still overextending your arm, try this: Stand close enough to a wall that a correctly executed punch stops just an inch or two short of hitting it. I promise you: You won't hit that wall more than a few times before you know where to stop.

- Depending on the punch, step, pivot, or lean into it with every part of your body from your head to your toes. That means you want to always look in the direction you're punching. Be sure to turn your head, shoulders, upper body, hips, knees, and feet that way too.

- Breathe with the punch. Exhale at the point of impact, inhale on the recovery.

- Give each punch a clear, definite destination—both going out and coming back. Find an external target to aim for. Just as important, have an internal visualization you can call on to maintain focus. I always think of my fists as my children: one is my daughter, Shellie, the other is my son, Billy, Jr. Just as I would never send my children on a journey without a map or directions, I never fire a punch without knowing where it's going and bringing it back with equal focus, power, and speed. You'll find that as you progress through Tae-Bo, the recovery action helps pick up the momentum that helps drive the next punch or next move.

- Keep your head up. You may have noticed that boxers and even some people in the videos punch with their chins down in a more guarded position. That's fine if you're a trained boxer, but if you're not, I want to see that head up so your chin is parallel to your shoulders—no higher or lower.

- Keep both shoulders down. If you don't come to Tae-Bo with a strong, well-developed upper body, you might be using your shoulder to pull up your arm instead of making your arm muscles do the work. This is a very common mistake, and if you're making it, you're bound to feel it sooner or later. Rather than risk injury or develop poor technique, check yourself in the mirror. If this is a problem, work on isolating the correct arm muscles.

- To make it easier for you to learn, the punches are always broken down into several parts. However, in the Tae-Bo Workout, we execute punches in one count, not two. In other words, it isn't "one" to punch and "two" to recover. It's "one" (punch, recover), "two" (punch, recover), "three" (punch, recover), and so on.

- If you find yourself falling off the count, be sure you're counting correctly and check your technique. Remember that snake I talked about before: always coiled and ready to strike. If you relax out of position on recovery—by letting too much of your weight shift to your heels or your back leg or by letting your guard down—you'll always be behind. Playing catch-up in your Workout sets off a vicious cycle of rushing, which results in poor technique, and poor technique not only gives you less of a workout but increases your risk of injury.

- Think of each punch as your fist pointing out the direction for your body to follow, and then make sure your body keeps up.

The Jab and the Cross: What Makes the Difference?

If you're new to Tae-Bo, you may have trouble telling a Jab from a Cross. Depending on the angle you're seeing them from, they can look very similar. You want to understand the differences so when the exercise or combination calls for one or the other, you're doing the right punch and not some in-between variation that combines them.

Their differences are detailed below, but here are a few quick ways to tell them apart:

- In a Jab, your leading foot is on the same side as your punch. So for a Left Jab, your left foot leads; for a Right Jab, your right.

- This is exactly opposite of your positioning for a Cross. There, you lead with the foot opposite of the side that's punching. So for a Left Cross, your right foot leads; for a Right Cross, your left.

- While both punches "cross" the body, they do it differently. In a Jab, the punching fist travels nearly straight out from the shoulder to a point of contact about a fist-width to the opposite side of center. So a Left Jab would make contact a fist-width right of center; a Right Jab would make contact a fist-width left of center.

- In a Cross, the path from your body to the point of impact is a more pronounced diagonal. Here the point of contact is the area directly in front of the shoulder opposite the side you're punching from. But since you're pivoting your whole body into this punch, and your opposite shoulder is turning away from the punch in the process, that puts your point of contact just about parallel to the opposite shoulder.

- You can visualize the differences in terms of a clock. If you're facing straight ahead and direct center is 12:00, picture a Left Jab at 1:00 to 1:30 and a Right Jab at 10:30 to 11:00. A Left Cross would land somewhere around 2:00 to 2:30 and a Right Cross somewhere between 9:30 and 10:00.

- One way you can test how well you're pivoting into the Cross and how well you're positioning your Jab is to try a two-punch combination: Left Jabs then Right Cross (or Right Jabs then Left Cross). You'll know you're pivoting correctly when the reach of your Cross exceeds the reach of your Jab. If it doesn't, then you're probably not turning your shoulders and hips far enough into the Cross.

You can make your punches more challenging by:

- doing them in double-time
- adding more reps
- adding more reps in double-time

You can do more reps of your punches by:

- doing them a little slower
- taking an eight-count break to shift to movement not concentrated in your arms—for instance, marching, jumping jacks, standing ab work—then returning to your punches

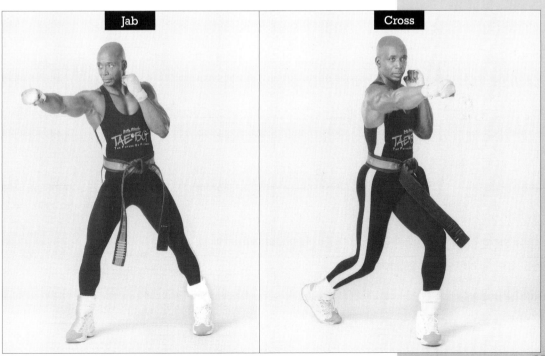

Jab

Cross

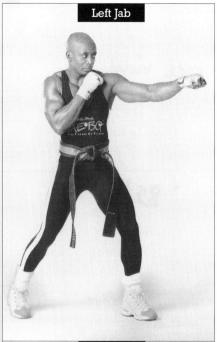

Left Jab

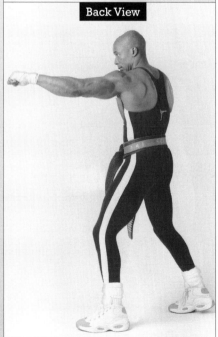

Back View

THE JAB

Of the four punches you'll be doing in Tae-Bo, the Jab is the only one that's not designed to knock an opponent out. In boxing, the Jab is called a setup punch, because it usually sets an opponent up for the real punch that follows. Remember this when you're doing the Jab, because while all the punches should be lightning-fast, the Jab connects a bit faster and a little lighter. I also say it's like the mosquito that distracts the opponent while you deliver the real punch, usually a Cross.

Most of the time in Tae-Bo, the Jab travels in an almost straight line out from your shoulder to the point of contact. As with all other punches, your point of contact is two to three inches short of full extension. I say "an almost straight line," because even though a Jab can look like it's traveling straight ahead, the point of contact is really about a fist-width to the opposite side of center. In other words, a Left Jab stops at a point about a fist-width right of dead center in front of you. A Right Jab stops at a point about a fist-width left of dead center in front of you.

In some Tae-Bo combinations, you will see variations on the straight forward Jab. You might jab to the side, or corner to corner in a shuffle/punch combination. Even though the direction is different, the technique is the same.

The Left Jab

1 Start from the Left Side Stance with your hands up in guard position.

2 With your left fist, punch out toward a point about a fist-width's distance right of center. Hold your abs tight and turn your shoulders, waist, and hips slightly to the right while you pivot your right foot with your heel up, so your weight moves forward to your left leg with the punch.

3 Recovering the punch, momentarily shift some weight from your left front leg to your right back leg as you return to the start position. Make sure you're still bending both knees slightly and not straightening your legs.

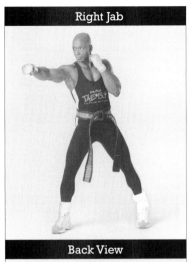

Right Jab

Back View

The Right Jab

1 Start from the Right Side Stance with your hands up in guard position.

2 With your right fist, punch out toward a point about a fist-width's distance left of center. Hold your abs tight and turn your shoulders, waist, and hips slightly to the left while you pivot your left foot with your heel up, so your weight moves forward to your right leg with the punch.

3 Recovering the punch, momentarily shift some weight from your right front leg to your left back leg as you return to the start position. Make sure you're still bending both knees slightly and not straightening your legs.

What's Wrong with This Picture?   *The Jab*

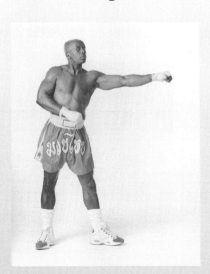

X *I'm punching straight out from my shoulder so the punch lands directly in front of my shoulder instead of a fist-width away from center.*

X *My left arm is fully extended.*

X *My right hand is not in the guard position. I can't be as physically or mentally aware as I should be. Not only am I not protecting myself as I punch, but keeping my arm down will make it harder for me to recover my punch.*

X *My feet are both planted, limiting my mobility, holding back my punch, and putting stress on my back and my knees.*

THE CROSS

The Cross is exactly what it sounds like: a punch that crosses your body to hit a target parallel to the opposite shoulder. The key to a powerful Cross is pivoting your entire body behind the punch.

The Left Cross

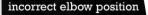
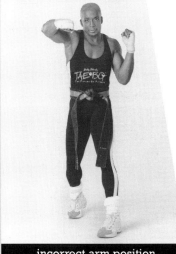

1 Start from the Right Side Stance with your hands up in guard position. With your left foot, take a step back so that your left foot is about a shoulder's-width distance behind but still parallel to your right foot.

2 Visualize your target: across your right shoulder about two to three inches short of full extension.

3 As you punch, lift your left heel, pivot to the right, and use your hips, waist, and shoulders to deliver the punch. Your right leg should be slightly bent, and your weight should shift forward to your right leg as you complete the punch.

4 Recover your left arm, making sure your body follows the same path back to the start position.

The Right Cross

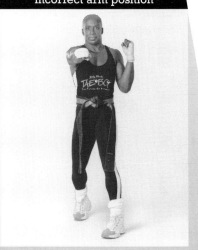

1 Start from the Left Side Stance with your hands up in guard position. With your right foot, take a step back so that your right foot is about a shoulder's-width distance behind but still parallel to your left foot.

2 Visualize your target: across your left shoulder about two to three inches short of full extension.

3 As you punch, lift your right heel, pivot to the left, and use your hips, waist, and shoulders to deliver the punch. Your left leg should be slightly bent, and your weight should shift forward to your left leg as you complete the punch.

4 Recover your right arm, making sure your body follows the same path back to the start position.

Right Cross

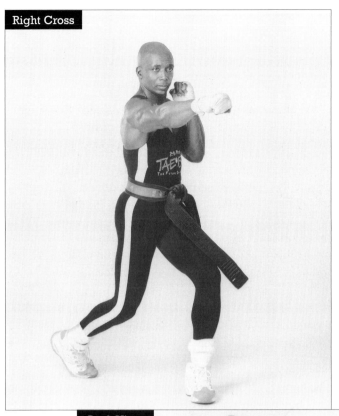

Back View

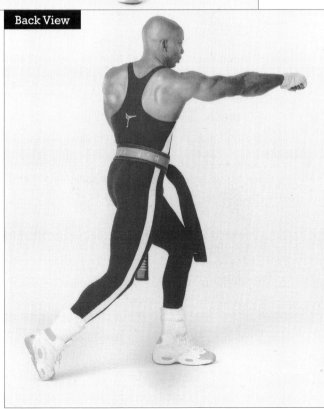

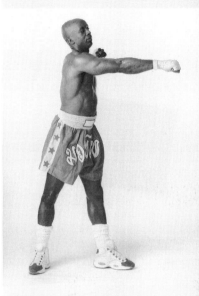

What's Wrong with This Picture?

The Right Cross

- ☒ My elbow is far too high.
- ☒ I've let my left guard hand get too far from my body.
- ☒ My elbow is fully extended and my arm is straight.
- ☒ My right foot isn't pivoting, and as a result, I'm not turning in to the punch but working against it.

155

THE CROSS WITH GUARD

Any time you execute a technique that uses reciprocal motion—that is, two parts of your body moving simultaneously in opposite directions—strive for the smoothest, most fluid motion you can achieve. Keep your technique sharp, while at the same time blurring the lines where one motion starts and the other begins. This should look like one continuous movement with no stops.

The Left Cross with Guard (Open-Handed)

1. Start from a Right Side Stance with your left, punching arm up in the guard position and your right arm slightly bent but extended straight out from your shoulder with your hand open, palm out, and fingers up. Eighty percent of your weight should be on your rear (left) leg and the rest concentrated in the ball of the right foot.

2. You'll be punching across your right shoulder, two or three inches short of full extension. You will be working both arms simultaneously, retracting your right guard as you execute the left punch, then extending your right guard outward as you recover the Left Cross.

The Right Cross with Guard (Open-Handed)

1. Start from a Left Side Stance with your right, punching arm up in the guard position and your left arm slightly bent but extended straight out from your shoulder with your hand open, palm out, and fingers up. Eighty percent of your weight should be on your rear (right) leg; the rest is in the ball of the left foot.

2. As in the Right Cross, you'll be punching across your left shoulder, two or three inches short of full extension. You will be working both arms simultaneously, retracting your left guard as you execute the right punch, then extending your left guard outward as you recover the Right Cross.

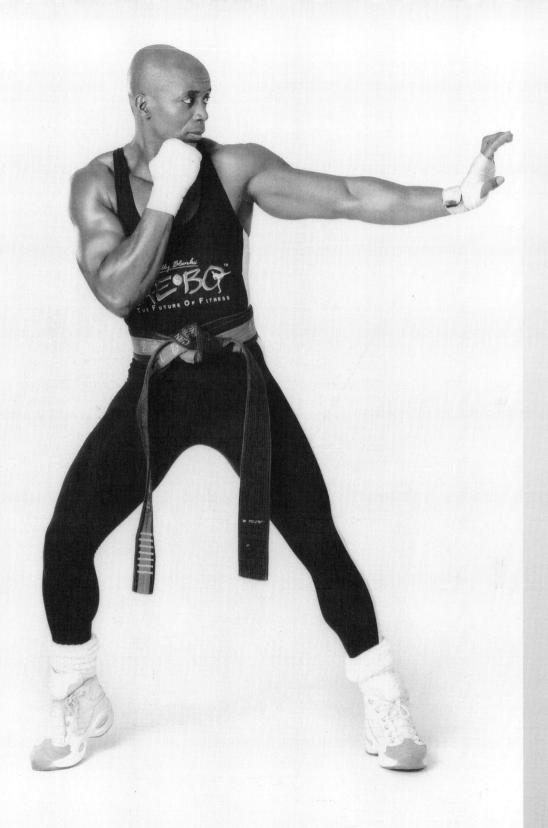

THE HOOK

The first few times you see it, the Hook may not look that different from a Cross. In both of them, you punch toward your opposite shoulder. The big difference is in the route your fist and body follow to reach the point of impact. For a moment, forget about punching straight ahead, as you do to Jab, or diagonally across, as you do to Cross. In the Hook, you'll be sending your punch along a route that traces a quarter circle from your guard to a target point directly in front of you, about sixteen inches from your chest. If your punching arm were a hand on a clock, your Right Hook would travel backward (counterclockwise) from 3:00 to 12:00; your Left Hook would travel forward (clockwise) from 9:00 to 12:00.

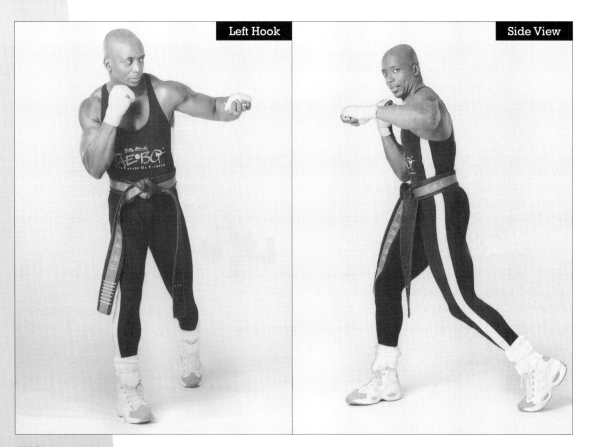

Left Hook

Side View

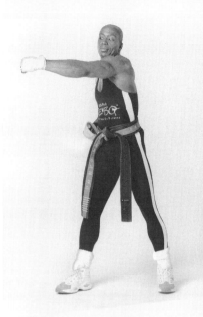

To correctly execute this punch, you must bring your elbow up so it's at the same level as your fist and just a few inches below your shoulder. You can keep your elbow from flying out of position by visualizing it traveling along an upside-down "L" that begins at your rib cage and ends in front of your punching shoulder. Your movement should be controlled, as if you had a string tying your upper arm to your rib cage. At the point of impact, try to concentrate your energy into a split-second thrust that puts your full force into the punch.

The Left Hook

1. Start from the Horse Stance, with your hands up in guard position. Your weight is distributed evenly between both legs.

2. Lift your left arm at the shoulder, so your left elbow and left fist are level. Visualize your fist traveling along that quarter-circle, and pivot both feet, making sure that your left knee and your left hip are following the same path. Stop two to three inches short of full extension.

3. Retract your fist, making sure that your elbow follows the same upside-down "L" pathway back.

The Right Hook

1. Start from the Horse Stance, with your hands up in guard position. Your weight is distributed evenly between both legs.

2. Lift your right arm at the shoulder, so your right elbow and right fist are level. Visualize your fist traveling along that quarter-circle, and pivot both feet, making sure that your right knee and your right hip are following the same path. Stop two to three inches short of full extension.

3. Retract your fist, making sure that your elbow follows the same upside-down "L" pathway back.

What's Wrong with This Picture?

The Left Hook

- ☒ I'm stuck in a Forward Stance because I'm centering my weight on my heels instead of on the balls of my feet.

- ☒ My poor stance is making it impossible for me to pivot. And without pivoting, I can't put any force behind my punch.

- ☒ I'm punching straight out from my body instead of tracing a quarter-circle from my punching shoulder to my target.

- ☒ My punching arm is fully extended, risking elbow injury.

- ☒ I'm not looking in the direction of my punch.

- ☒ I've dropped my right hand, so I have no guard up.

159

THE UPPERCUT

The secret to successful execution of the Uppercut lies in visualizing the path your fist will travel from your guard to the point of impact. This time, your fist will start from your lower rib cage and reach a point about a foot out from your face, close to chin level. Be sure that as you punch, your fist is moving in a slightly rounded curve, like it did in the Hook, not moving straight up nor at an angle. Visualize tracing the round side of a backward "C," or a crescent, from the bottom to the top. Do not bend your wrists.

In the instant before each punch, you want to use your bent knees to dip down very slightly—just an inch or two—then spring back up with the punch (but without fully straightening either leg or locking your knees) and turning your punching shoulder into the punch as you exhale. To keep this momentum and correct form when doing a series of repetitions on either side, be sure you return completely to the start position. Think of each return as a windup for the next punch. And keep that punch smooth and controlled. You don't want to accidentally hit yourself in the face.

The Left Uppercut

1 Start from the Horse Stance with your hands in a guard position, but parallel to your shoulders instead of under your chin.

2 As you pivot both feet, turn your left knee, your left hip, your waist, and your left shoulder to your right and into the punch. At the same time, you want to be sure your right knee is slightly bent so you can give your punch that upward thrust. At the point of impact, your left arm will be two to three inches short of full extension and your left fist will be about twelve inches out from your face.

3 Return completely to the start position.

The Right Uppercut

1 Start from the Horse Stance with your hands in a guard position, but parallel to your shoulders instead of under your chin.

2 As you pivot both feet, turn your right knee, your right hip, your waist, and your right shoulder to your left and into the punch. At the same time, you want to be sure your left knee is slightly bent so you can give your punch that upward thrust. At the point of impact, your right arm will be two to three inches short of full extension and your right fist will be about twelve inches out from your face.

3 Return completely to the start position.

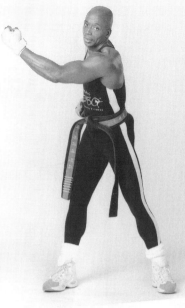

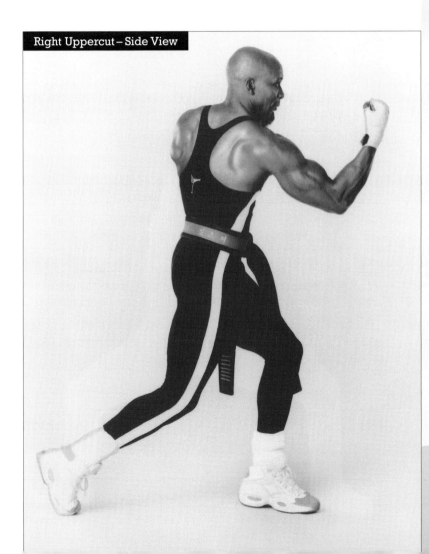

Right Uppercut – Side View

What's Wrong with This Picture?

The Left Uppercut

X *I'm not pivoting with both feet into the punch. Instead, I'm only twisting at the waist, which is bound to strain my knees, my hips, and my back.*

X *Standing straight with my weight in my heels and my knees locked, I can't move sideways or up. My punch is dead.*

X *My Uppercut is completely without direction and is traveling out from my body instead of out, up, and in again.*

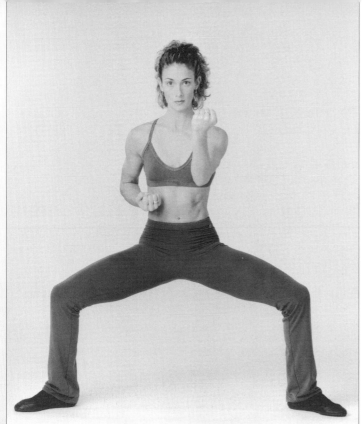

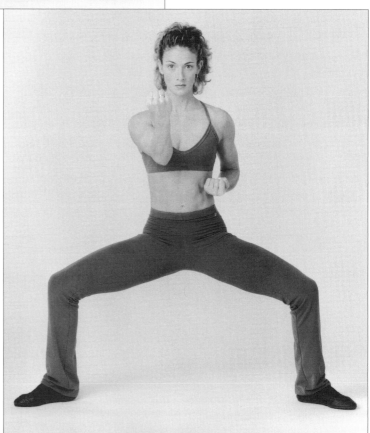

ALTERNATING UPPERCUTS

Alternating Uppercuts can be challenging, because your body is making both a pivoting, twisting motion and rising slightly upward behind the punch. The key to giving this move rhythm and flow is to make sure that your feet and your arms are always either moving or ready to move. Think for a minute about what happens when you swim. Say you're doing a crawl or a back-stroke. You don't stroke with your right arm, pause, then begin the next stroke with your left. You keep both arms in motion constantly. Whenever you're alternating punches or kicks, the same principle applies. As your left fist reaches the point of impact, your right fist should begin moving forward, and they should pass each other at a midpoint in between.

Concentrate your weight on the balls of both feet at all times. If you're sure that you're fully turning your body correctly, you can also tap with the pivoting toes. Some people find this makes changing direction easier.

THE SPEEDBAG IN A HORSE STANCE

Here it may look—and feel—like your arms are doing all the work. But to develop good Speedbag technique you have to concentrate on the correct positioning of your other nonmoving body parts, especially your abs and your shoulders. You'll see the results in tighter abs and more clearly defined shoulders and arms.

■ *Really strive to make your arm motions as smooth as pedaling a bicycle. You want your motion to be so smooth and continuous, no one can see where one punch ends and the next one begins.*

■ *Think like a boxer: You want to hit your imaginary bag with the top of your knuckles, not the flat of your fist or your knuckle joints.*

■ *Many people find their stance is more comfortable if they relax enough to bounce slightly on their legs. Try this if you feel any tightness in your lower back. Make sure, however, that you're not so relaxed that your knees extend beyond your toes.*

■ *Keep your abs tight and your rib cage high. Leaning back just slightly and exhaling thoroughly will help you.*

1 Start from the Horse Stance. Facing forward, bend your elbows and raise your fists so the thumb side faces you, the palm side faces down, and they're both level with your chin, six to eight inches in front of you. Your right fist should be an inch or two above your left.

2 Beginning with your right fist, punch in a small, tightly controlled circle away from and then back toward you. Follow with your left. Both fists should be moving continuously and aligned so that when you look at your fists in motion, your speed and positioning create the illusion of one fist, not two.

3 Count normally, bearing in mind that you should be executing about four full circles (two with each fist) per count in regular time and about eight in double-time.

4 As your speedbag technique speeds up and gains momentum, you may have to concentrate to keep your abs tight and your shoulders down and level. This is especially true after a couple of repetitions, when you begin to tire. This is where it helps to bounce a little on your legs—but not on your knees. Now your legs can act like shock absorbers, making it easier to stabilize your abs and your shoulders.

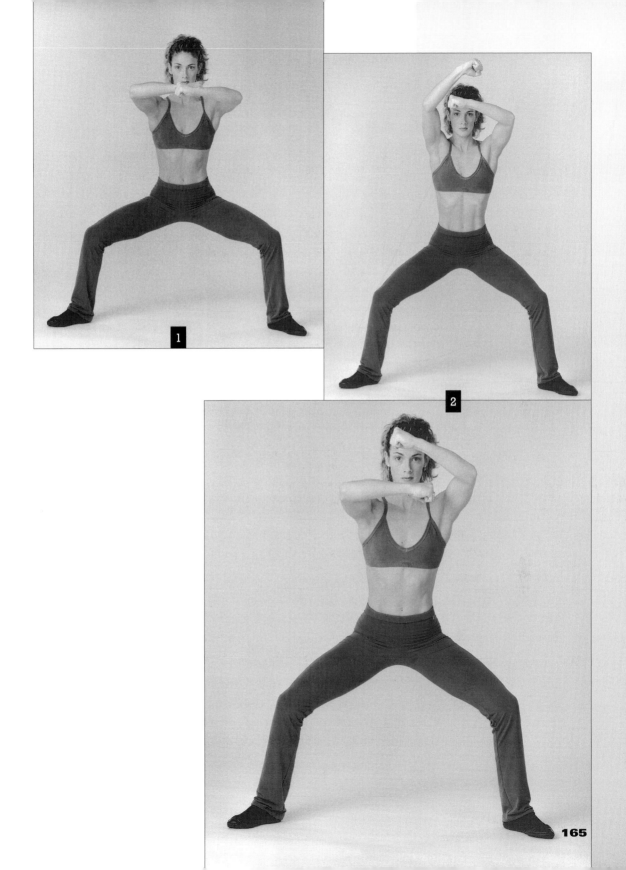

THE SPEEDBAG IN A MODIFIED HORSE STANCE

The Speedbag in a Modified Right Horse Stance

1 From the Horse Stance, pivot right with both feet so you're facing right. Bend your elbows and raise your fists so the thumb side faces you, the palm side faces down, and they're level with your chin, six to eight inches in front of you. Your right fist should be an inch or two above your left.

2 Beginning with your right fist, punch in a small, tightly controlled circle away from and then back toward you. Follow with your left. Both fists should be aligned and moving continuously so when you look at your fists in motion, your speed and positioning create the illusion of one fist, not two.

3 Count normally, bearing in mind that you should be executing about four full circles (two with each fist) per count in regular time and about eight in double-time.

4 As your speedbag technique speeds up and gains momentum, you may have to concentrate to keep your abs tight and your shoulders down and level. This is especially true after a couple of repetitions, when you begin to tire. This is where it helps to bounce a little on your legs. Your knees should be slightly bent. Now your legs can act like shock absorbers, making it easier to stabilize your abs and your shoulders.

The Speedbag in a Modified Left Horse Stance

1 From the Horse Stance, pivot left with both feet so you're facing left. Bend your elbows and raise your fists so the thumb side faces you, the palm side faces down, and they're level with your chin, six to eight inches in front of you. Your left fist should be an inch or two above your right.

2 Beginning with your left fist, punch in a small, tightly controlled circle away from and then back toward you. Follow with your right. Both fists should be aligned and moving continuously so when you look at your fists in motion, your speed and positioning create the illusion of one fist, not two.

3 Count normally, bearing in mind that you should be executing about four full circles (two with each fist) per count in regular time and about eight in double-time.

4 As your speedbag technique speeds up and gains momentum, you may have to concentrate to keep your abs tight and your shoulders down and level. This is especially true after a couple of repetitions, when you begin to tire. This is where it helps to bounce a little on your legs. Your knees should be slightly bent. Now your legs can act like shock absorbers, making it easier to stabilize your abs and your shoulders.

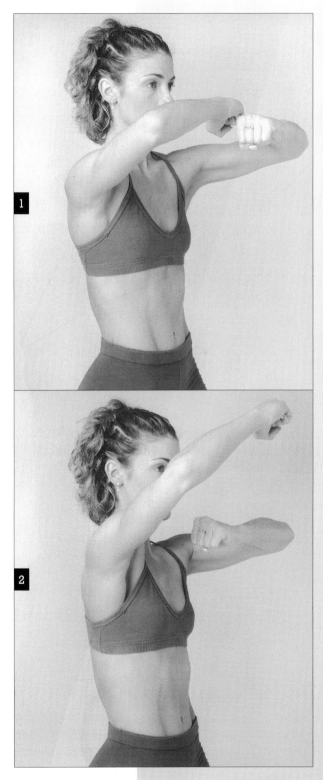

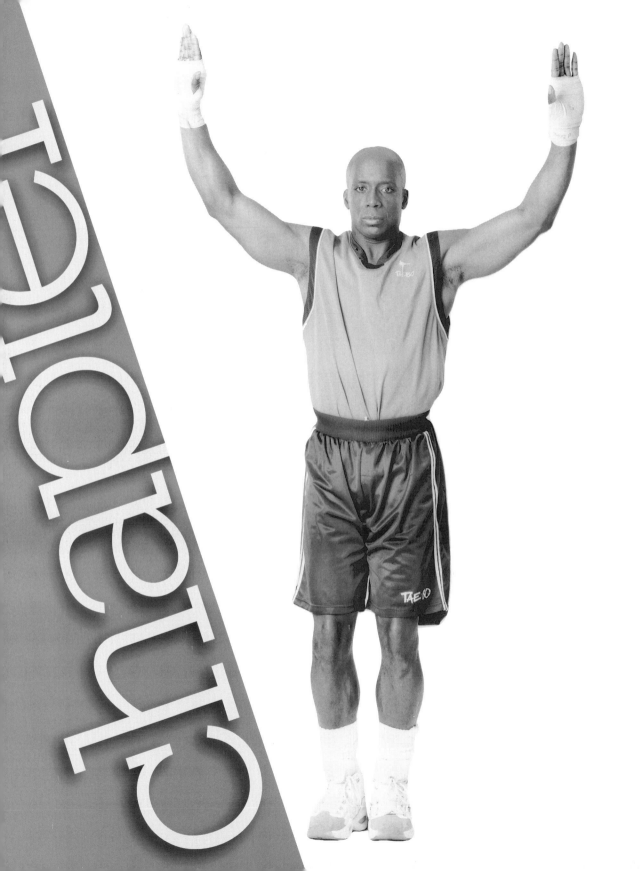

eight

Troubleshooting Your Technique

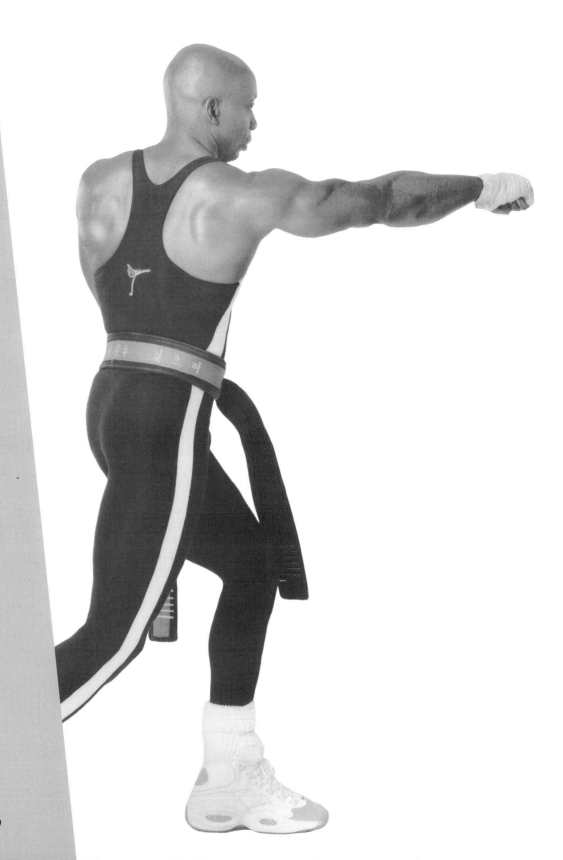

When I created Tae-Bo, I made sure to use movements that most people could learn easily and do safely. The details of technique, the tips on breathing, positioning, balance, reciprocal force, and many other subjects are here for you to learn and to apply to your Workout. Ultimately, you are responsible for yourself. No one else can possibly know how your Workout feels to you. This is why I believe self-awareness is so important. I know I've said it before, but it bears repeating: Almost every injury can be traced back to a lack of awareness and focus and the sloppy technique that usually follows.

Doing Tae-Bo, you may find yourself doing things you either haven't done in a while or have never done before. Because it's an intensive, full-body workout, you may feel muscles you didn't even know you had before. And that's all good. There's nothing wrong with feeling that burn or coming off the floor a little sore all over for a day or two. It's your body, so you need to know not only when and how to push yourself through that fire, but also when to hold back. In most cases, a specific problem can be traced back to poor technique. If you're giving your Tae-Bo Workout all you've got, you can expect to feel a little general soreness all over. This is especially true if you haven't worked out in a while or are using muscles you haven't used much before. But the kind of muscle soreness that comes from regular muscle fatigue should be something you continue feeling as long as you're doing Tae-Bo. I'm not going to tell you no pain, no gain. Working out should never be painful. But if you're working out and never feeling that your muscles haven't been at least challenged, you've hit a plateau and you're not putting as much into—or getting as much out of—your Workout as you could.

The chart that follows is intended to help you work through any difficulties you might be having. Remember, though, you know your body best. If you frequently experience discomfort in the same spot on your shoulder when delivering a particular punch, the problem probably is your technique. Use the chart to help you correct your technique and see how it feels a few days later. If the discomfort persists, or if you experience pain in a specific area when you're doing other moves as well, consult your doctor. The good news is that for most people, an awareness of how they're moving and a correction in their technique is enough to keep them going.

PROBLEM	POSSIBLE CAUSE	TO IMPROVE YOUR TECHNIQUE...
BASIC FORWARD STANCE, SIDE STANCE, HORSE STANCE, SIDE HORSE STANCE		
Discomfort in knee	You may be bouncing too hard on your legs	Bend your knees slightly
	You may be bending your knees too deeply, so they extend beyond your toes	Don't bend so deeply
	You may have your weight concentrated in your knees	Concentrate your weight in your heels and your glutes (butt)
Discomfort in shin	You may be placing excessive pressure on your knees	Concentrate your weight in your heels and your glutes (butt)
Discomfort in lower back	You may be standing with your upper body hunched forward and over	Stand tall with your upper body straight and your abs tight
Discomfort in neck and back	You may be standing with your upper body hunched forward and over	Stand tall with your upper body straight and your abs tight
	You may be tensing your muscles	Relax your muscles so that they're coiled and ready to move but not tight
PIVOTING		
Discomfort in ankle, knee, or hip	You may not be fully turning on the balls of your feet	Focus on turning completely on the balls of your feet; be sure the pivoting heel is up off the floor
	Your shoes or your feet may be catching on the floor surface	Try either working on a floor that is not carpeted, or one that is covered with a very smooth, low-pile carpet; work out barefoot; switch to shoes with smoother soles
Discomfort in lower back	You may not be turning into your punch with your whole body	Focus on turning your whole body in one motion; be sure you're not turning your legs while your hips stay square, or pivoting on your feet, but not turning at the knee

PROBLEM	POSSIBLE CAUSE	TO IMPROVE YOUR TECHNIQUE...
BOUNCING FOOTWORK		
Discomfort in ankles, shins, or knees	Instead of moving up and down smoothly, you may be moving back and forth with too much force and using your knees, shins, and ankles as "brakes" to stop yourself	Concentrate on moving your whole body and softly bouncing; try making it one continuous motion instead of surging forward and stopping, then jerking backward and stopping, then surging forward again
KNEE RAISES, FRONT AND SIDE		
Discomfort in lower back	You may be hunching over as you raise your leg	Stand straight with your rib cage high and your abs tight. Remember: You're bringing your knee to your stomach, not your stomach to your knee
	You may be letting your foot land too heavily between lifts or letting your foot drop	Instead of fully stepping back down between raises, just let your foot touch the floor lightly. Whatever you do, be sure every movement is controlled
	You may be doing all the lifting with your lower back instead of your hip flexors	Focus on using your hip flexor to lift your knee to your belly button
Discomfort in the hip flexor	You may be swinging your leg out from the hip instead of lifting it by first using your abductors	Stand tall and stabilize your upper body and use your abductors to lift your leg
Discomfort in standing leg, usually around the knee	You may be locking your knee or bouncing too hard when you lift	Keep your standing leg slightly bent at the knee, with most of your weight concentrated in the heel of your standing leg
SIDE KNEE RAISE		
Discomfort in abdominal oblique muscles	You may be dropping your leg instead of recovering it with full control	Concentrate on recovering your leg with control

PROBLEM	POSSIBLE CAUSE	TO IMPROVE YOUR TECHNIQUE...
ALTERNATING FRONT KNEE RAISES		
Discomfort in the hip flexor	You may be raising your hip instead of raising your knee and using your hip flexor to raise your knee	Keep your hips square and use your hip flexors to pull your knee up
PUNCHES		
Headache, discomfort in neck	You may be using your shoulders to hold up your arms or letting your hands drop below chest level. Either puts pressure on your neck and creates muscle tension	Concentrate on using your arm muscles to support your arms, and keep your hands in the proper guard position
	You may be pulling your neck away and/or your head back as you punch	Be aware that you're doing this and focus on keeping your head and upper body forward even as you punch
Discomfort, or pinching sensation in your trapezius (upper back and neck area)	You may be tensing up your neck and shoulder muscles while you're in your guard and as you punch	Remember that the muscles that should be working the hardest are in your arms
	You may not be using a full range of motion when you punch	If you're cutting your movements short, you're going to tense up your muscles. Use the full range of motion for each punch. If you're too tired to do that, move on and do something else for a few minutes, then get back into the Workout
Discomfort in the elbow and/or shoulder	You may be fully extending your arm at the point of impact	Never fully extend your arm when you punch. Be sure your elbow is bent enough so the point of impact is two to three inches short of full extension

PROBLEM	POSSIBLE CAUSE	TO IMPROVE YOUR TECHNIQUE...
Discomfort in the elbow	You may be lifting your arm and punching only from the elbow down	Punch with your whole arm, your shoulder, and your whole body
Discomfort or cramping in your punching hand or arm	You may be squeezing your fist too tightly	Relax your fist, then, following the instructions on page 149, make a correct fist that's firm but not tense
Discomfort in your back and shoulders, particularly in combinations	You may be hunching your shoulders, rounding your back, or punching from your elbows	Watch your posture. Remember that your upper body should stand like a pillar. Keep your head up, rib cage lifted, abs tight, and your legs slightly bent

SPEEDBAG

PROBLEM	POSSIBLE CAUSE	TO IMPROVE YOUR TECHNIQUE...
Discomfort in lower back	You may be hunching over as you punch	Focus on keeping your upper body straight and your weight centered in the back of your legs and in your heels, concentrating on the glutes and the hamstrings
Discomfort in shoulder and neck	You may be using your shoulder muscles to "hold up" your arms	Stop and relax your shoulders and your neck. Bring your arms up into position again, but focus on making your arm muscles do the work and keeping your shoulders and neck relaxed

FRONT KICK

PROBLEM	POSSIBLE CAUSE	TO IMPROVE YOUR TECHNIQUE...
Discomfort in the hip flexor	You may be swinging your leg outward from the hip	Practice doing the Front Knee Raise by doing several repetitions, then concentrate on raising your knee before you kick
	You may not be lifting your knee to your belly button before you kick	Practice kicking above a coffee table, a bench, or another object. This will help "remind" you to pick up your knee. If you don't, you'll hit your foot on the object

PROBLEM	POSSIBLE CAUSE	TO IMPROVE YOUR TECHNIQUE...
Discomfort in the hip flexor (cont.)	You may be letting your kicking foot fall back to the floor	Be sure that when you recover your leg after the kick, your leg follows the same path back to the start position that it took going out
Discomfort in the lower back	You may be hunching forward	Be sure that your upper body is straight and that you're focusing your weight on your back, supporting leg
Discomfort in the knee	You may be fully extending your leg when you kick	Never fully extend your leg in any kick. Be sure that your point of impact is two to three inches short of full extension

SIDE KICK AND ROUNDHOUSE KICK

PROBLEM	POSSIBLE CAUSE	TO IMPROVE YOUR TECHNIQUE...
Discomfort or cramping in your feet	You may be trying to keep your balance by "gripping" the floor with your toes	Check your body position at every point. Be sure your feet are turned properly, you're fully pivoted, and you've found your balance before you raise your knee to kick
Discomfort in the kicking knee	You may be extending your kicking leg too far out	Never fully extend your leg in any kick. Be sure that your point of impact is two to three inches short of full extension
Discomfort in your lower back	You may be extending your kicking leg too far out	Never fully extend your leg in any kick. Be sure that your point of impact is two to three inches short of full extension
Discomfort in your standing leg	You may be locking your knee	Be sure that your standing leg is bent slightly at the knee

PROBLEM	POSSIBLE CAUSE	TO IMPROVE YOUR TECHNIQUE...
Discomfort in the lower back	You may not be turning your standing foot in the proper direction	Always be sure that your standing leg is positioned so that the heel of that foot is facing the same direction that you are kicking. That means that the toes of your standing leg will be pointed away from the kick

BACK KICK

PROBLEM	POSSIBLE CAUSE	TO IMPROVE YOUR TECHNIQUE...
Discomfort in the lower back	Your starting position may be wrong	Be sure that you're leaning forward from the hip, pushing your butt out, and keeping your weight correctly distributed
	You may be kicking out too hard or fully extending your leg	Never fully extend your leg in any kick. Be sure that your point of impact is two to three inches short of full extension. Also, be sure that when you kick back, you're leading the kick with your heel, not your toe
Discomfort in knee of kicking leg	You may be fully extending your leg when you kick	Never fully extend your leg in any kick. Be sure that your point of impact is two to three inches short of full extension

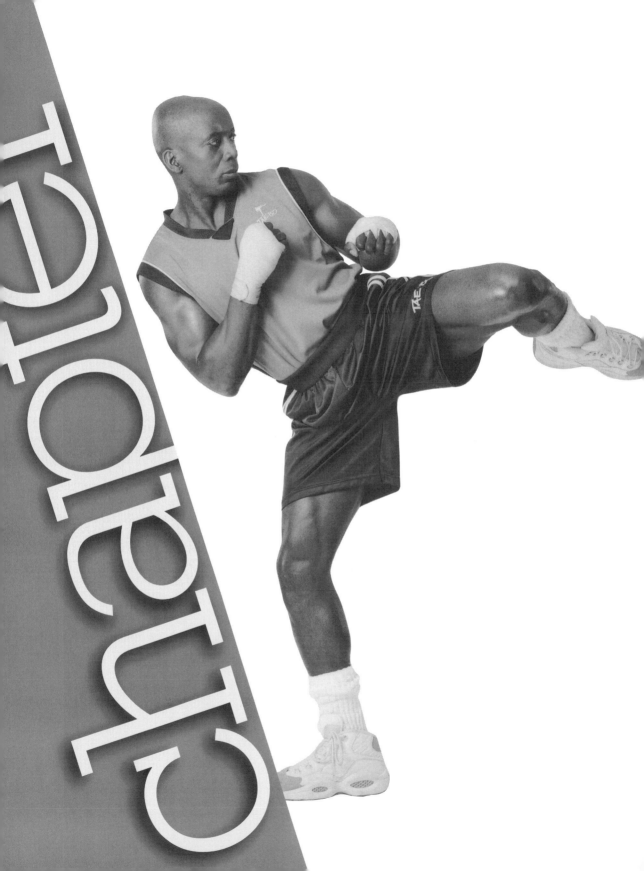

nine

Mastering Your Tae-Bo Workout

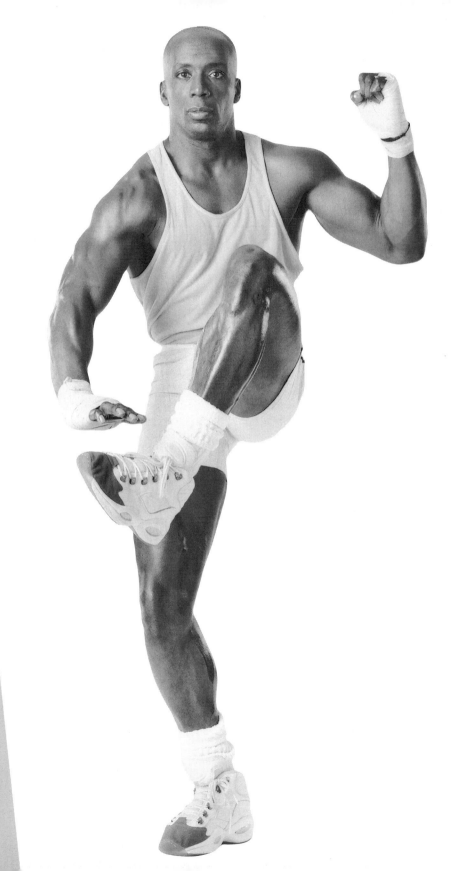

For many people, the Combinations are the most challenging, exciting, and energizing part of Tae-Bo. This is really what it's all about, because Combination work forces you to bring together everything you've learned about Tae-Bo—balance, positioning, technique, and focus—and apply it with complete awareness of what you're doing and why.

The success of a Combination depends on every piece being in place. Your stances and starting positions, the execution of your punches and kicks, the direction you're moving and facing, the strength of your recoveries—each of these can make or break your Combination. A sloppy recovery will leave you a split-second behind going into the next move, for instance. A poor return position may make it impossible for you to make your next move without difficulty.

As you do Combinations, especially in the beginning, be aware of your weak points and how they can detract from the overall Combination. Work on those moves and techniques that are giving you the most trouble. Be especially on the lookout for poor recovery. A leg that just drops after a kick or an arm that falls after a punch are often behind Combinations that never seem to get going with any rhythm or flow. Incomplete pivoting is also another weak spot, particularly in those Combinations that require you to move quickly into and out of kicks and punches or make quick changes in direction. The answer: Practice, practice, practice. And then practice some more.

Combinations also depend on keeping the right rhythm and finding that flow that makes you feel like one move is pushing you right into the next. A good Combination feels more like a dance than a group of specific moves executed in quick succession. You can't dance if you don't have the rhythm, and that brings us back to counting. This is particularly true if you're watching a videotape while working out or working out in a class or with a buddy. If you fall out of time or get lost, the first thing you'll probably do is look around to see what someone else is doing. That's only natural, but it's one of the worst things you could do. Instead of watching others and trying to jump back into the beat, close your eyes and feel the

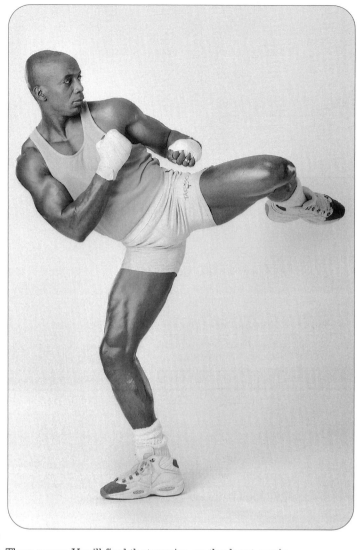

count from the inside. Then move. You'll find that you're on the beat again instead of being slightly off. And your movements will come from what your mind is telling your body to do, not from imitating someone else. Think back to what I said about every move being a fresh print: crisp, clear, and sharp. Imitating what you see someone else do is like tracing: The outlines may be almost right—you'll be kicking when everyone else does—but the clarity, the sharpness, and the purpose won't be there. People who move by imitating are so distracted by watching someone else that their technique always suffers. If you know how to execute a move and you're having trouble keeping up with Combinations, close your eyes, turn your back on the television, or look away from your buddy.

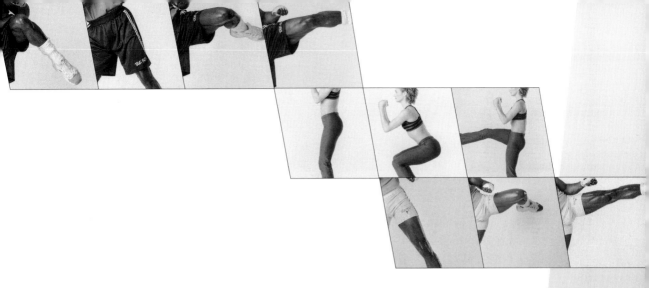

The Principles of Combination Work

- ◘ Tae-Bo works from the inside out, and so should you. You need to have absolute control over your movements, and that requires complete focus. Train yourself to think more about what you're feeling and what you're doing than the sights and sounds that can distract you.

- ◘ Keep every movement as clean and as sharp as you can. If poor technique in one part of the Combination is dragging the whole Combination down, take time to work on it separately.

- ◘ Complete recovery is essential for Combinations, even though individual moves inside the Combination may end in positions slightly different than they would if you were just doing reps of the same move. Here's where your awareness and focus come into play.

- ◘ Don't move between thoughts, but train your mind to think ahead to the next move while still completing the one you're in. This is especially true when your next move requires a change in position or stance that is not the one you usually recover the current move in.

- ◘ If you feel that you can't execute every move in a Combination smoothly or comfortably, be creative and modify it. You can work at half-time, kick or punch once instead of twice, kick or raise your knee to lower than stomach level, or take two counts to pivot instead of one and eliminate a move that follows. As long as you have good technique and are using the full range of motion in everything you do, you're still in the Workout.

- ◘ Practice as much as you can, including outside the Workout, until you master the Combinations. Combination work is not only great for your body, it's a lot of fun.

FRONT KNEE RAISE/CROSS

This is a simple Combination, but watch your breathing. Since you exhale on both the Knee Raise and the Cross, be sure to inhale between moves. The Knee Raise works your abs and your glutes, while the Cross works your arms, your upper body, and your waist. This is done in two counts: Knee Raise ("one"), Cross ("two").

Right Front Knee Raise/Left Cross

1 Stand in a Forward Stance, with both hands up in an open guard. Take a single step back with your right foot; your left, supporting leg will be slightly bent.

2 Do a Right Front Knee Raise. Exhale as you tighten your abdominal muscles and bring your right knee up to your stomach. Touch your right foot with your left hand. Be careful not to bend at the waist or twist from the left down toward your knee. Your knee is coming up to your stomach and your hand; your stomach shouldn't be going down to meet your knee.

3 Bring your right foot down so your heel touches down on the area of the floor that was directly under your lifted right knee. As you assume a Right Side Stance, inhale and pivot to the right as you execute a Left Cross and exhale. Be sure as you shift your weight right that your right knee is bent, but not so deeply that it covers your right toes.

4 Recover the Left Cross, pivoting back to the start position.

5 Once you recover the Left Cross, shift your weight back to your left leg, which will be the supporting leg again as you repeat the Combination with a Right Front Knee Raise. Continue for two to three sets of 8 reps.

Left Front Knee Raise/Right Cross

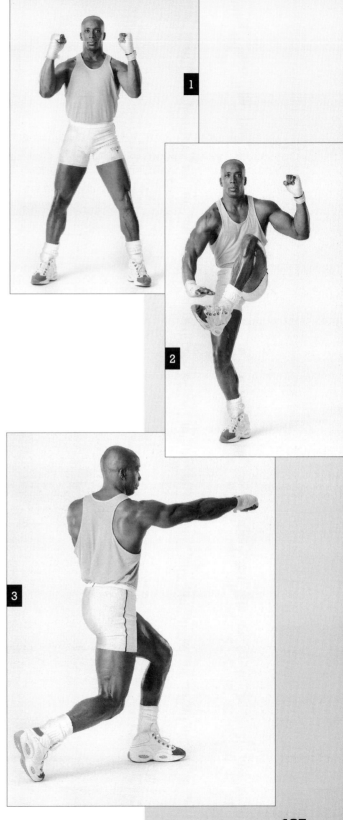

1 Stand in a Forward Stance, with both hands up in an open guard. Take a single step back with your left foot; your right, supporting leg will be slightly bent.

2 Do a Left Front Knee Raise. Exhale as you tighten your abdominal muscles and bring your left knee up to your stomach. Touch your left foot with your right hand. Be careful not to bend at the waist or twist from the right down toward your knee. Your knee is coming up to your stomach and your hand; your stomach shouldn't be going down to meet your knee.

3 Bring your left foot down so your heel touches down on the area of the floor that was directly under your lifted left knee. As you assume a Left Side Stance, inhale and pivot to the left as you execute a Right Cross and exhale. Be sure as you shift your weight left that your left knee is bent, but not so deeply that it covers your left toes.

4 Recover the Right Cross, pivoting back to the start position.

5 Once you recover the Right Cross, shift your weight back to your right leg, which will be the supporting leg again as you repeat the Combination with a Left Front Knee Raise. Continue for two to three sets of 8 reps.

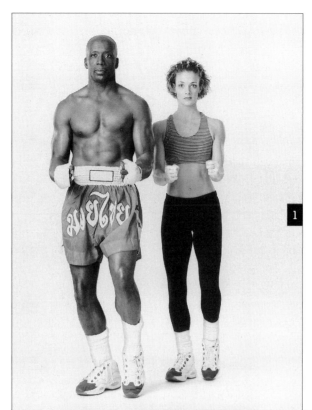

1

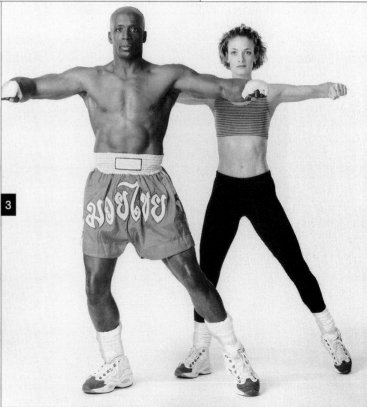

3

SHOULDER FLY/ TOE TOUCH

This simple Combination is a great workout for your shoulders, back, biceps, and triceps. The secret is to keep your abs tight and your torso as straight as a pillar. Concentrate on your arm and leg movements, and when doing a series of reps on one side, let your moving foot touch down lightly. Each rep is done in one count.

1 Start facing front in a Forward Stance with your arms bent and your fists held at waist level and in front of your body.

2 Bend your knees a few inches more, putting your weight into your heels, and make sure your bent knees are not covering your toes.

3 Raise both arms up to shoulder level, keeping your elbows bent. This is a smooth, tightly controlled movement. At the same time, lightly touch out at least a foot to your left or right with that foot; your toe, not your whole foot, should touch the floor.

4 Return to the start position, being careful to keep the arm and the leg movements in sync. Repeat this Combination for two to three sets of 8 reps on each side.

SQUAT/FRONT KICK

This Combination really works your glutes, so don't be surprised if you find yourself tiring after just a few sets. You can do more reps by not squatting as deeply, but the more deeply you squat and the longer you can stick with this, the quicker you'll see results. Each Squat-Kick counts as "one."

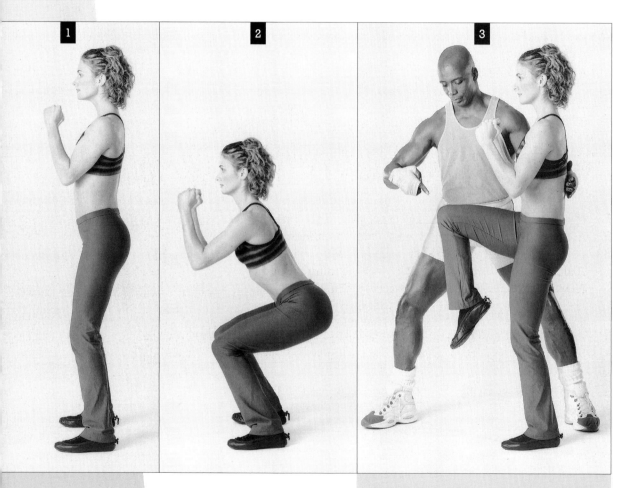

Notice that Shellie is completing a Front Knee Raise before she extends her leg out into the Front Kick. Taking care to complete each movement before starting the next one will help you get more out of your Workout.

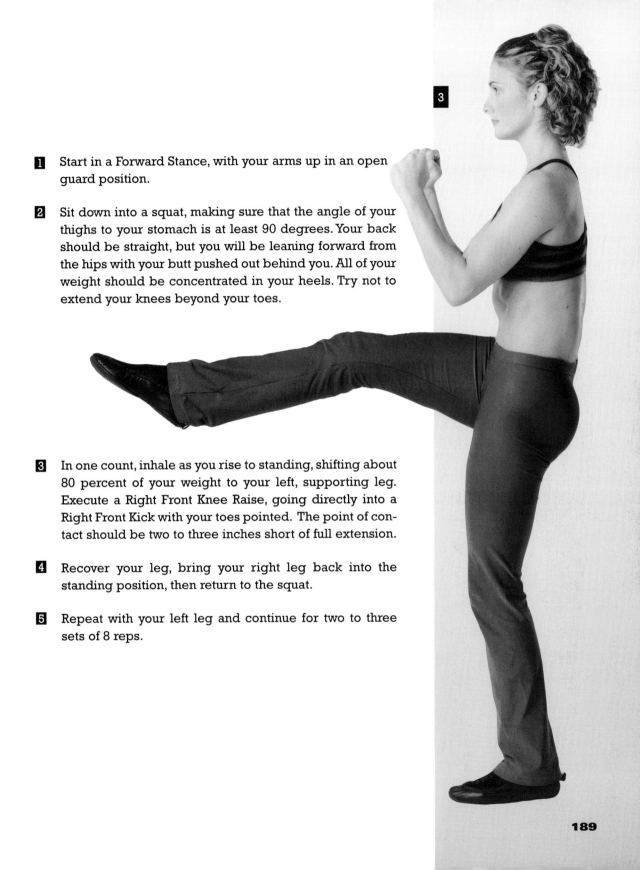

3

1 Start in a Forward Stance, with your arms up in an open guard position.

2 Sit down into a squat, making sure that the angle of your thighs to your stomach is at least 90 degrees. Your back should be straight, but you will be leaning forward from the hips with your butt pushed out behind you. All of your weight should be concentrated in your heels. Try not to extend your knees beyond your toes.

3 In one count, inhale as you rise to standing, shifting about 80 percent of your weight to your left, supporting leg. Execute a Right Front Knee Raise, going directly into a Right Front Kick with your toes pointed. The point of contact should be two to three inches short of full extension.

4 Recover your leg, bring your right leg back into the standing position, then return to the squat.

5 Repeat with your left leg and continue for two to three sets of 8 reps.

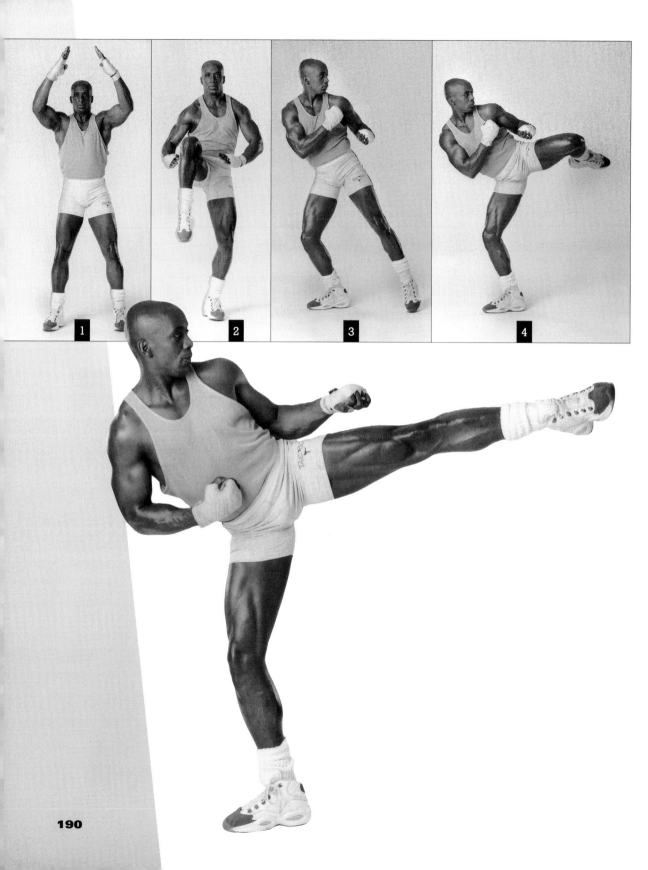

FRONT KNEE RAISE/ ROUNDHOUSE KICK

This Combination is done in two counts: Knee Raise ("one"), Kick ("two"). The trick to doing this Combination is to keep it flowing by replacing one foot with the other as you go from the Knee Raise into the Roundhouse Kick.

Right Front Knee Raise/Left Roundhouse Kick

1 From a Forward Stance, raise both hands over your head, with your palms facing inward.

2 In one count, do a Right Front Knee Raise as you bring your hands down to touch your knee.

3 As you finish the Knee Raise, make sure you are pivoting into position for the Roundhouse Kick, so that your toes are facing to the right and your heels to the left for the Left Roundhouse Kick.

4 With about 80 percent of your weight now shifted to your right leg, execute a Left Roundhouse Kick. Make sure that your right leg is slightly bent.

5 Recover the kick, bringing your left leg down and pivoting your feet forward so you are ready for the Right Front Knee Raise that begins the next rep.

6 Repeat this Combination for two to three sets of 8 reps.

Left Front Knee Raise/Right Roundhouse Kick

1 From a Forward Stance, raise both hands over your head, with your palms facing inward.

2 In one count, do a Left Front Knee Raise as you bring your hands down to touch your knee.

3 As you finish the Knee Raise, make sure you are pivoting into position for the Roundhouse Kick, so that your toes are facing to the left and your heels to the right for the Right Roundhouse Kick.

4 With about 80 percent of your weight now shifted to your left leg, execute a Right Roundhouse Kick. Make sure that your left leg is slightly bent.

5 Recover the kick, bringing your right leg down and pivoting your feet forward so you are ready for the Left Front Knee Raise that begins the next rep.

6 Repeat this Combination for two to three sets of 8 reps.

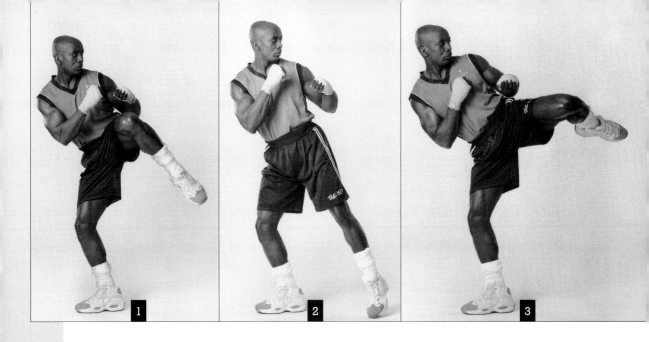

DOUBLE SIDE KNEE RAISE/ ROUNDHOUSE KICK/CROSS

This entire Combination should be completed over four counts: Knee Raise ("one"), Knee Raise ("two"), Kick ("three"), Cross ("four"). The trick to staying on count is to move quickly and surely into the pivoted chamber position for the Roundhouse Kick and then to recover that quickly to go into the Cross. When you do reps of this, think of the Double Side Knee Raises as a bit of a rest before the second, more challenging half of the Combination.

Double Left Side Knee Raise/Left Roundhouse Kick/Right Cross

1 From a Forward Stance, take a single step straight back with your left foot. Raise both hands over your head, with your palms facing inward. In one count, shift most of your weight to your right, supporting leg, and execute a Left Side Knee Raise as you bring your hands down to touch your knee.

2 Fully recover your left leg (don't let it just drop) and repeat. After the second Side Knee Raise, recover your foot again, but make sure that as it hits the floor, you have both feet together and you are pivoting, with toes to the right

and your heels facing left for the Left Roundhouse Kick.

3 With about 80 percent of your weight now shifted to your right leg, execute a Left Roundhouse Kick.

4 Recover the kick, bringing your left leg down, a little in front of your right and turning your left foot so that it's again facing forward, then execute your Right Cross. Come back to the start position for the Left Side Knee Raise that begins the next rep.

5 Repeat this Combination for two to three sets of 8 reps.

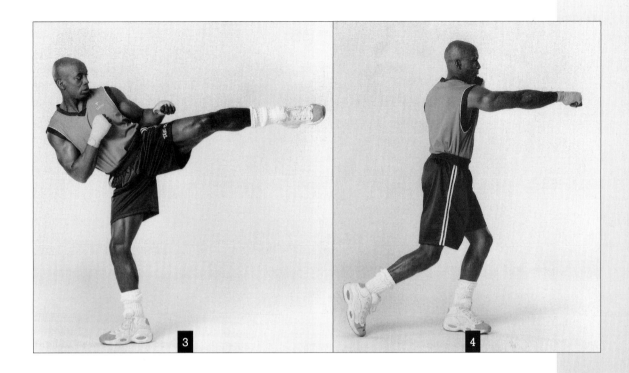

Double Right Side Knee Raise/Right Roundhouse Kick/Left Cross

1 From a Forward Stance, take a single step straight back with your right foot. Raise both hands over your head, with your palms facing inward. In one count, shift most of your weight to your left, supporting leg, and execute a Right Side Knee Raise as you bring your hands down to touch your knee.

2 Fully recover your right leg (don't let it just drop) and repeat. After the second Side Knee Raise, recover your foot again, but make sure that as it hits the floor, you have both feet together and you are pivoting, with your toes to the left and your heels facing right for the Right Roundhouse Kick.

3 With about 80 percent of your weight now shifted to your left leg, execute a Right Roundhouse Kick.

4 Recover the kick, bringing your right leg down, a little in front of your left and turning your right foot so it's again facing forward, then execute your Left Cross. Come back to the start position for the Right Side Knee Raise that begins the next rep.

5 Repeat this Combination for two to three sets of 8 reps.

JUMPING JACK / JAB

The key to this simple Combination is making sure that your arms come down in the Jumping Jack in the correct position to punch and to guard. Note that your legs do not come together when your arms go down; they stay wide to provide a solid stance for the Jab. Start the Jumping Jack with your fists made and with full awareness and control over your arm muscles. Don't let them flap upward like you did in gym class as a kid. Even this should be a controlled motion. And this one is fast: You Jab on every count, so the Jumping Jack has to move.

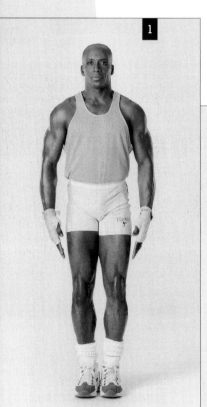

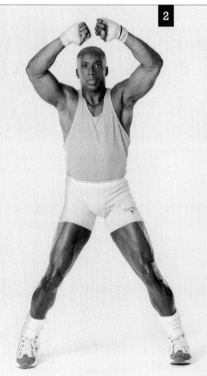

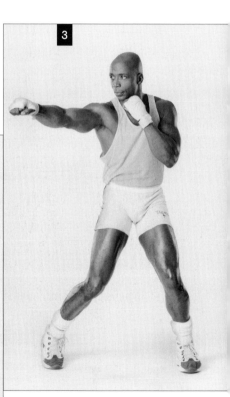

1. Stand facing forward, with your feet together, parallel and flat on the floor. Your arms should be down at your sides.

2. As you raise your arms up over your head for the first part of the Jumping Jack, open your legs so they're at least a foot wider than shoulder-distance apart. As you lift your arms, they should be slightly bent at the elbow (not straight) and your hands should be in the correct fist position.

3. Bring your arms down, with your left hand in a guard and your right ready to punch. Execute a Right Jab, making sure to pivot into the punch from your right foot, knee, and hip.

4. At the moment of impact, reposition your right foot so that it's facing front for the Jumping Jack.

5. As you raise your arms up over your head for your second Jumping Jack, open your legs so that they're at least a foot wider than shoulder-distance apart. As you lift your arms, they should be slightly bent at the elbow (not straight) and your hands should be in the correct fist position.

6. Bring your arms down, with your right hand in a guard and your left ready to punch. Execute a Left Jab, making sure to pivot into the punch from your left foot, knee, and hip.

7. At the moment of impact, reposition your left foot so that it's facing front for the Jumping Jack. Repeat for two to three sets of 8 reps.

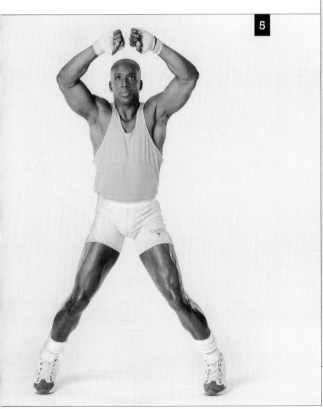

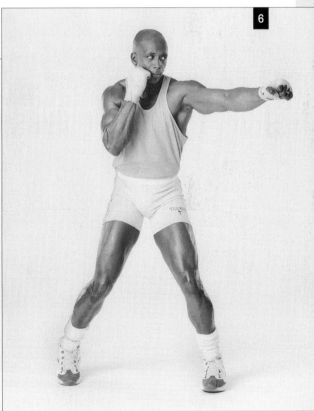

FRONT KNEE RAISES/ FRONT KICK/ JUMPING FRONT KICK

The Jumping Front Kick is the first Tae-Bo move most students see once and say, "I'll never be able to do that." But you can, and you will. It's very simple, and nothing that you haven't done before in Tae-Bo. In the simplest terms, a jump happens whenever both feet leave the ground at the same moment. The only difference between a jump and a step is the timing. The Jump Kick comes a split-second sooner than you'd expect. That's what gives it the height, and the look and the feel of something much more difficult.

Now, this can be tricky. And if you find yourself always doing a regular Front Kick instead of jumping, try to "reset" your timing. It's all timing. Remember: Everything you do in Tae-Bo is based on skills you've already learned. If you take your time and work at it, you can do it too.

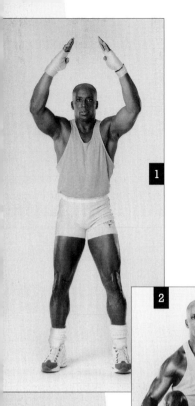

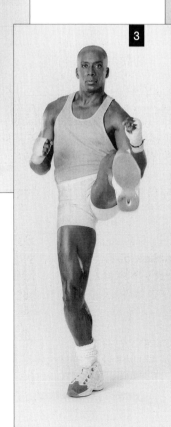

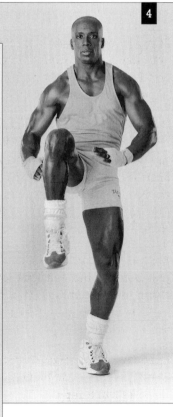

196

Right Front Knee Raises/Left Front Kick/Jumping Left Front Kick

1 From a Forward Stance, raise both hands over your head, with your palms facing inward.

2 In one count, shift most of your weight to your left, supporting leg, and execute a Right Front Knee Raise as you bring your hands down to touch your knee.

3 Recover your right leg, and as you bring it down, shift your weight for the next move, the Left Front Kick. Execute this kick and remember to stop the kick two

to three inches short of full extension. Bring your hands down to a regular open guard position.

4 Repeat the Right Front Knee Raise, but just before your right foot touches back down, use the momentum from the lift on that side to start the Jumping Left Front Kick.

5 Execute the Jumping Left Front Kick. Return to start position. Repeat for two to three sets of 8 reps.

Left Front Knee Raises/Right Front Kick/ Jumping Right Front Kick

1 From a Forward Stance, raise both hands over your head, with your palms facing inward.

2 In one count, shift most of your weight to your right, supporting leg, and execute a Left Front Knee Raise as you bring your hands down to touch your knee.

3 Recover your left leg, and as you bring it down, shift your weight for the next move, the Right Front Kick. Execute this kick and remember to stop the kick two to three inches short of full extension. Bring your hands down to a regular open guard position.

4 Repeat the Left Front Knee Raise, but just before your left foot touches back down, use the momentum from the lift on that side to start the Jumping Right Front Kick.

5 Execute the Jumping Right Front Kick. Return to start position. Repeat for two to three sets of 8 reps.

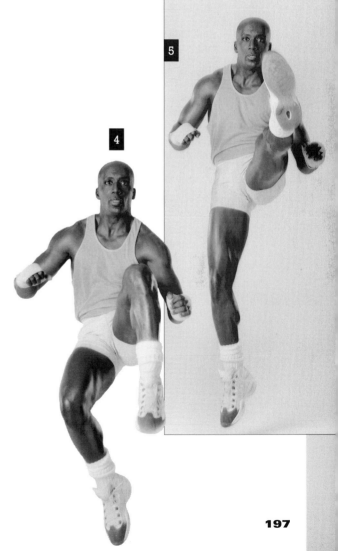

Here's a Combination that looks simple yet seems to trip some people up. When students do have problems, it's usually due to poor technique and overdoing some of the movements. They tend to step too widely and reach too far with the punch instead of keeping all the movements quick, tight, and close to the body. There are a few secrets to success with this Combination:

- *Look and move in the direction you're punching.*

- *When you step as you Jab, keep the step in sync with the Jab. I see some students fall into a pattern of stepping then Jabbing, stepping then Jabbing. Or Jab, step, Jab, step, Jab, step. Or they're moving their front foot, then their back instead of moving both together. A whole class doing that looks like a bunch of galloping horses. You don't want that up-and-down, stop-start kind of motion. You want it smooth and fast. If you're having trouble with the timing, break that move out separately, and practice coordinating your step with your Jab.*

- *When you're stepping, pick up your knees and keep the steps shorter rather than longer. Long steps or lunges (which you should not be doing) will slow you down and throw off your timing. Try to keep your step as short and as quick as your punch. It might help if you say, "Pop-pop-pop" instead of counting. If you can only move a short distance in that time, then do that.*

- *When you finish the third Jab, think ahead: Your next move is a Cross from the opposite side. Get that guard hand ready to punch and that back leg set to pivot.*

- *As you deliver the Cross, keep standing tall. Some students tend to let their knees bend and their body weight drop, so it starts to look more like a lunge. Don't do that. It will slow your recovery and make it harder to start the next set of Jabs in the opposite direction.*

- *As you recover from the Cross, fully turn your entire body in the opposite direction. Be aware of your feet and your knees especially. Don't just turn your upper body and leave your legs behind. Make this shift in direction quick, clean, and complete.*

TRIPLE JAB/CROSS

Each punch/step is one count, so this entire exercise, done once on each side, should be completed over a single eight-count.

1 From a Left Side Stance, deliver a Left Jab as you take one step left. Notice that while you're moving to one side, you are not moving sideways. Both feet should be pointing to the left.

2 Repeat the Left Jab/step Combination two more times.

3 Still facing left, on "four" deliver a Right Cross. As you recover your arm, pivot completely so you're in a Right Side Stance and ready to move to the right.

4 Deliver a Right Jab as you take one step right. Notice that while you're moving to one side, you are not moving sideways. Both feet should be pointing to the right.

5 Repeat the Right Jab/step Combination two more times.

6 Still facing right, on "eight," deliver a Left Cross. As you recover your arm, pivot completely so you're in a Left Side Stance and ready to move to the left.

7 Repeat for two to three sets of 8 reps.

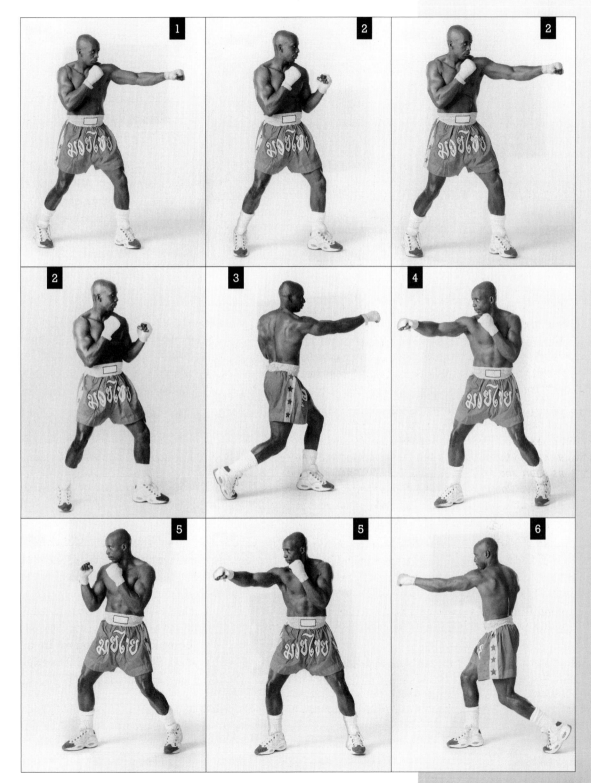

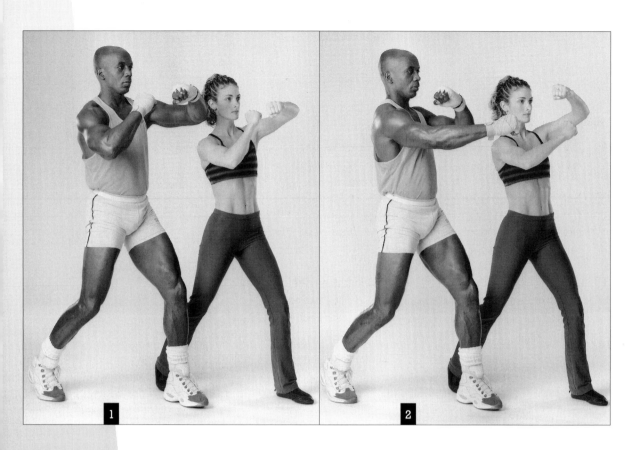

SPEEDBAG WITH JAB

This is great for your arm muscles and your abs, and it's simple to do. Each set is eight reps, with each Jab counting as one.

Left Speedbag with Left Jab

1 From a Left Side Stance, raise your arms for the Speedbag, with your left fist an inch or two above your right.

2 Beginning with your left fist, start the Speedbag, bearing in mind that you should be executing about four full circles (two with each fist) per count in regular time and about eight in double-time.

3 Execute three circles of Speedbag punches. After "three," pull your arms back to left guard postion, execute a quick Left Jab on "four," then resume the Speedbag. Repeat for two to three sets of 8 reps on your left.

Right Speedbag with Right Jab

1 From a Right Side Stance, raise your arms for the Speedbag, with your right fist an inch or two above your left.

2 Beginning with your right fist, start the Speedbag, bearing in mind that you should be executing about four full circles (two with each fist) per count in regular time and about eight in double-time.

3 Execute three circles of Speedbag punches. After "three," pull your arms back to right guard postion, execute a quick Right Jab on "four," then resume the Speedbag. Repeat for two to three sets of 8 reps on your right.

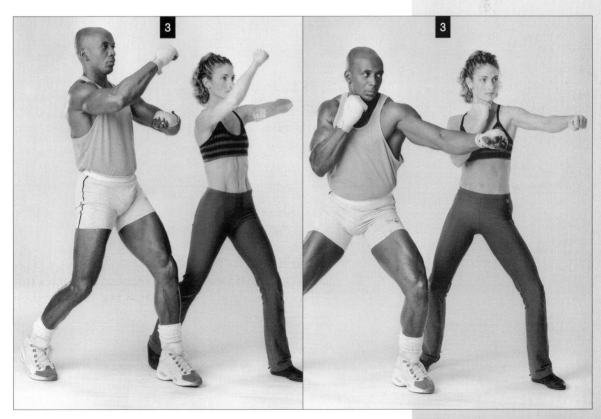

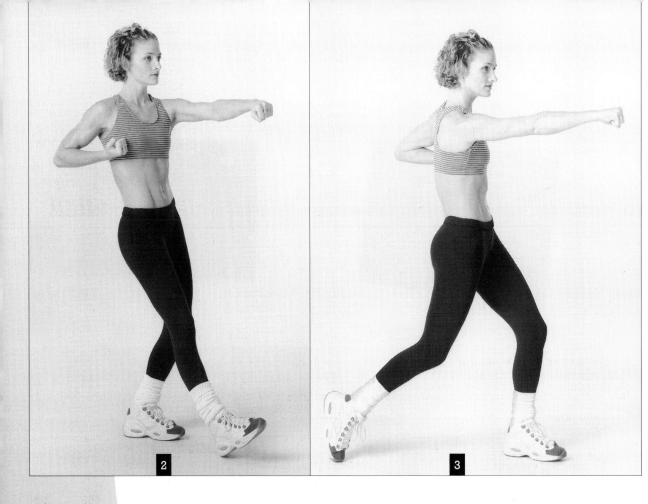

2

3

ALTERNATING
TOE-HEEL/PUNCH

This Combination may look complicated, but it's really a variation on movements we make every day when we're walking. Your supporting leg should always be slightly bent, and your punch should stop a few inches short of full extension. As you tap your heel and your toe, make it a sharp, clear movement. Don't let your feet drag. Each punch counts as one.

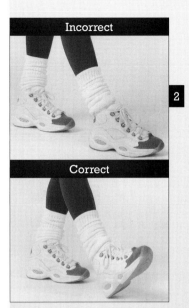

2

1 Stand with your feet facing forward, about hip-distance apart. Bend both arms at the elbows, make fists, and bring your elbows back until both fists are resting at your sides, just a few inches in front of and below your armpits. Your fists should be palms up.

2 As you execute a Left Jab (be sure to rotate your fist as you punch), extend your right foot, tapping the floor in front of you with your right heel.

3 As you recover the Left Jab, execute a Right Jab while tapping the floor behind you with your right toe.

4 Repeat on one side for two to three sets of 8 reps. Switch sides.

5 From the starting position, as you execute a Right Jab (be sure to rotate your fist as you punch), extend your left foot, tapping the floor in front of you with your left heel.

6 As you recover the Right Jab, execute a Left Jab while tapping the floor behind you with your left toe.

7 Repeat on one side for two to three sets of 8 reps.

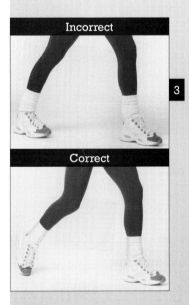

3

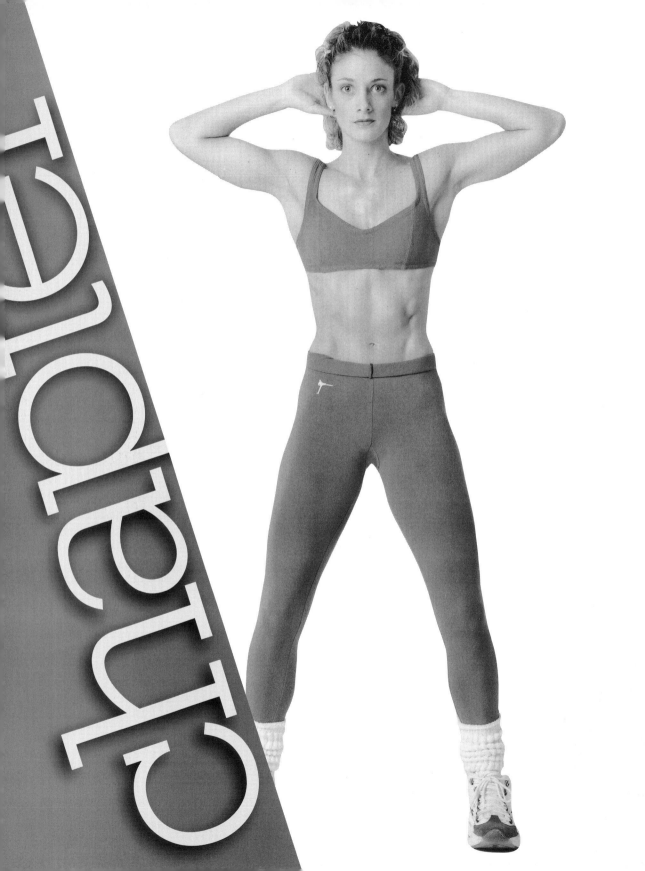

chapter

ten

Floor Work and Ab Work

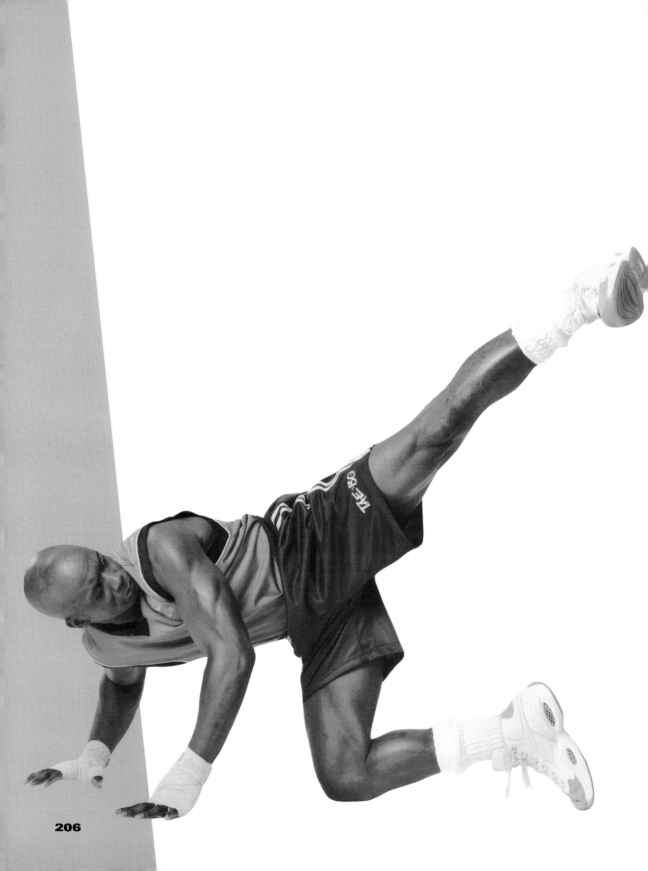

206

This part of the Tae-Bo Workout is the easiest to learn and the most challenging to do. Whenever it's time for Floor Work in a class, you can hear the groans. Even the most dedicated students let me know this is the part of the Workout they dread. But that's okay with me, because I designed it to be intense, demanding, and draining. If there's ever a time in your Workout when your will is really put to the test, this is going to be it. No matter how long you do Tae-Bo, you're never going to reach the point where you breeze through these. If you do, you should add more reps until you find yourself going through the fire again.

Now, for some people, what you just read would give them every reason to quit before they even started, to skip the Floor Work altogether. But you're different, because you're doing Tae-Bo. You know the value of having strong abdominals, tight glutes, and powerful thigh muscles. You know that you're going to see the results of every abdominal crunch and every leg lift—especially those few very last ones you complete through pure will. Improved stamina, sharper technique, effortless balance, and increased strength are great, invisible results. But there's even more: a flat stomach, defined waistline, firm butt, and fat-free thighs. Get on the floor! We've got work to do.

As you do these exercises, always remember to:

- Focus on the muscles you're working. Talk to yourself and to your body. Instead of moaning about the difficulty, cheer your body on for the great work you're doing.

- Keep every muscle you're working tight and controlled. You may not see a lot of movement in some of these exercises, but you should really feel every muscle you work.

- Remember to inhale on pulling moves (in this series of exercises, those are the rests between the moves that call for big muscle contractions), and to exhale on pushing moves (tightening your abdominals, lifting your legs).

- These exercises are designed to improve endurance and tone, so do as many reps as you can while maintaining good form. These exercises should bring on muscle fatigue and that good burn. Expect it, and when it happens, remind yourself of how much better you're going to feel and perform when you're done.

- Keep your mental guard up. All through Tae-Bo, I've told you to have an imaginary opponent. Make your fatigue and discomfort your opponents. Don't run away from them. Don't let them beat you. Whose Workout is this, anyway? Who's the boss? By now, I shouldn't have to tell you that you are.

- Even though you're not punching or kicking at an imaginary opponent, always maintain a focus point. If it helps you to have an opponent, make it the desire to stop. You can beat it!

The Floor Work

The Floor Work in Tae-Bo works the same muscles we use in kicks and combinations. The difference between working these muscles while you're kicking and in Floor Work is that balance is less of a problem when you're down on your hands and knees. Most people can do far more reps in Floor Work than they can do in kicks, and on the floor, you can usually raise your leg at angles and heights that would be far more difficult if you were standing.

For the five exercises that follow, always remember:

- When you're on your hands and knees, try to square your shoulders and your hips so that you're not bending at the waist or pushing one hip or shoulder out of line with the other.

- Keep your movements focused and smooth as well as fully controlled from start to finish. If you start to feel discomfort in your lower back, you may be throwing your leg or letting it drop.

- Keep your back comfortably straight, but not tense. Be careful not to arch your back when you raise your leg, or dip between your shoulders and your hips when you recover your leg.

- Try to keep your hands in exactly the same position: with your elbows slightly bent and your weight concentrated on your fingers and first knuckle joints (where your fingers meet your hands), not on your palms. Avoid having the palm of the hand on the side of your supporting leg flat against the floor while rising on the fingers of the other hand. This will cause you to lean to the side of the supporting leg and can cause stress in your back.

- When you raise your leg, don't shift all of your weight to the supporting leg. Also be sure that you're not leaning so hard into your supporting leg that the line between your knee and your hip isn't fairly straight. Leaning too far away from the lifting leg puts stress on your lower back and your supporting hip.

- Raise your leg as high as you can comfortably, but don't let fatigue stop you from pushing even further.

- Keep your head up. Always try to look in the direction your leg is moving, or at least keep your head up. Don't let your head hang.

- Tighten those abs! Make sure that when you do, you're not rounding your back.

- If you start to feel muscle fatigue, it's better to slow down and do fewer reps than to quit totally.

- As with any move in Tae-Bo, the recovery is as important as the actual kick. Never let your leg drop. Return to the starting position following the same path it took on the way out.

- Each raise or kick counts as "one."

- For the best results, try to do the Floor Work exercises in this order.

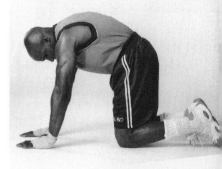

What's Wrong with This Picture?

Floor Work Starting Position

- **X** My back is arched instead of flat and straight. From this position, it would be very difficult to do the Floor Work without placing stress on my supporting leg and my back.

- **X** My palms are flat against the floor, which concentrates too much of my weight in my hands and arms instead of distributing it evenly between my arms and my legs. From this position, I'll be more likely to push forward when I lift my leg.

- **X** My head is hanging, which means I'm not looking where my body is moving and the weight of my head is pulling on my neck, upper back, and shoulder muscles.

BACK KICK

Right Back Kick

1 Position yourself on all fours, making sure that your hands, elbows, stomach, and knees are correctly placed as described above.

2 With your right foot flexed, raise your leg, leading the movement with your right foot, not your knee. As your right foot rises, it should remain a few inches higher than your right knee.

3 Execute a Back Kick, stopping a few inches short of full extension. Focus on pushing the heel of your foot upward, toward the ceiling instead of straight back behind you. Focus on isolating the muscles in your legs and your butt. Do not let your lower back swing upward on the kick.

4 In a smooth, controlled motion, bring your right leg back down to the start position. On the Back Kick, be especially careful not to let your foot drop suddenly. Repeat for two to three sets of 8 reps.

Left Back Kick

1 Position yourself on all fours, making sure that your hands, elbows, stomach, and knees are correctly placed as described above.

2 With your left foot flexed, raise your leg, leading the movement with your left foot, not your knee. As your left foot rises, it should remain a few inches higher than your left knee.

3 Execute a Back Kick, stopping a few inches short of full extension. Focus on pushing the heel of your foot upward, toward the ceiling instead of straight back behind you. Focus on isolating the muscles in your legs and your butt. Do not let your lower back swing upward on the kick.

4 In a smooth, controlled motion, bring your left leg back down to the start position. On the Back Kick, be especially careful not to let your foot drop suddenly. Repeat for two to three sets of 8 reps.

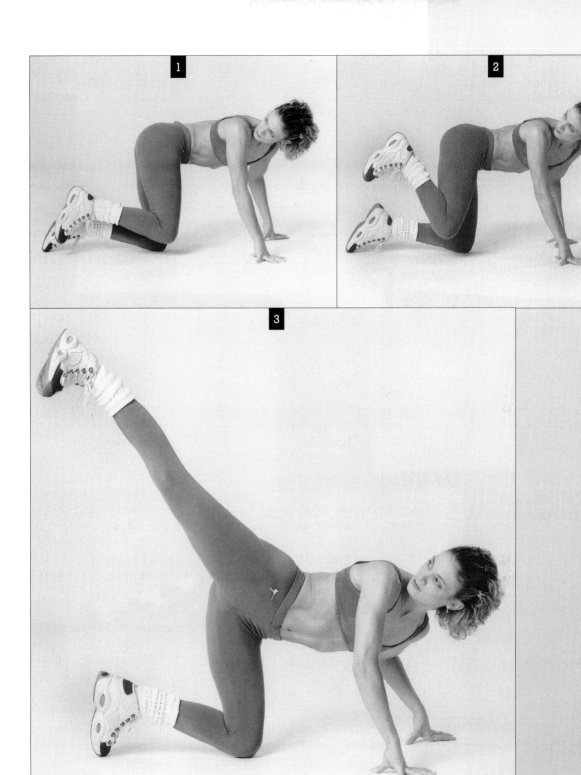

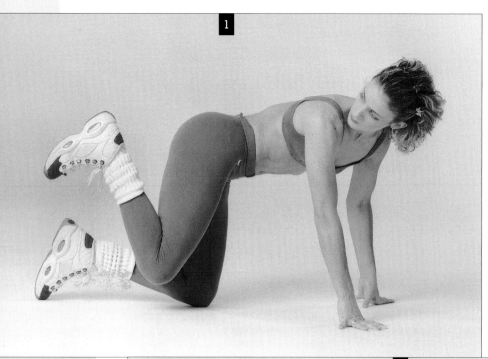

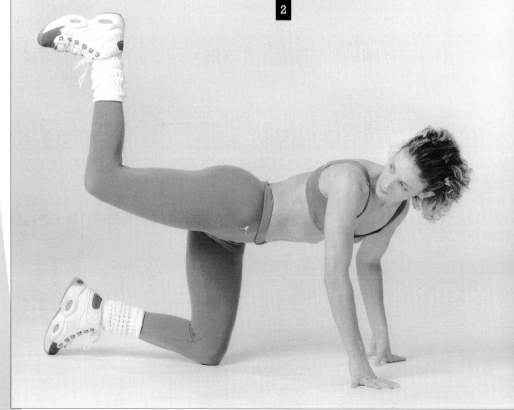

KNEE RAISE

Right Knee Raise

1 Position yourself on all fours, making sure that your hands, elbows, stomach, and knees are correctly placed as described above.

2 With your right foot flexed, raise your right leg straight up toward the ceiling until your knee reaches hip level. As you do, really squeeze your glutes to get the full effect.

3 In a smooth, controlled motion, return to the start position. If you're doing reps, try not to touch down. If you do touch down, keep your weight concentrated on your left leg. Repeat for two to three sets of 8 reps.

Left Knee Raise

1 Position yourself on all fours, making sure that your hands, elbows, stomach, and knees are correctly placed as described above.

2 With your left foot flexed, raise your left leg straight up toward the ceiling until your knee reaches hip level. As you do, really squeeze your glutes to get the full effect.

3 In a smooth, controlled motion, return to the start position. If you're doing reps, try not to touch down. If you do touch down, keep your weight concentrated on your right leg. Repeat for two to three sets of 8 reps.

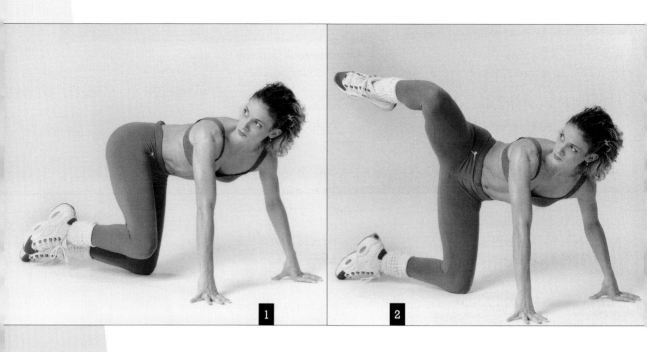

ROUNDHOUSE KICK

Right Roundhouse Kick

1 Position yourself on all fours, making sure that your hands, elbows, stomach, and knees are correctly placed as described above.

2 With your right toes pointed and your leg bent at the knee as shown, raise your right leg as close to parallel to the floor as you comfortably can.

3 Keeping your upper leg steady, execute a Roundhouse Kick to the side, about two to three inches short of full extension. At the point of impact, your instep should be facing toward your head.

4 Bring your right knee and your right foot back into position, so your upper leg is parallel to the floor. Your foot, knee, and hip should all be at the same level.

5 In a smooth, controlled motion, bring your right leg back down to the start position. If you're doing reps, try not to let your right knee touch down. Repeat for two to three sets of 8 reps.

Left Roundhouse Kick

1 Position yourself on all fours, making sure that your hands, elbows, stomach, and knees are correctly placed as described above.

2 With your left toes pointed and your leg bent at the knee as shown, raise your left leg as close to parallel to the floor as you comfortably can.

3 Keeping your upper leg steady, execute a Roundhouse Kick to the side, about two to three inches short of full extension. At the point of impact, your instep should be facing toward your head.

4 Bring your left knee and your left foot back into position, so your upper leg is parallel to the floor. Your foot, knee, and hip should all be at the same level.

5 In a smooth, controlled motion, bring your left leg back down to the start position. If you're doing reps, try not to let your left knee touch down. Repeat for two to three sets of 8 reps.

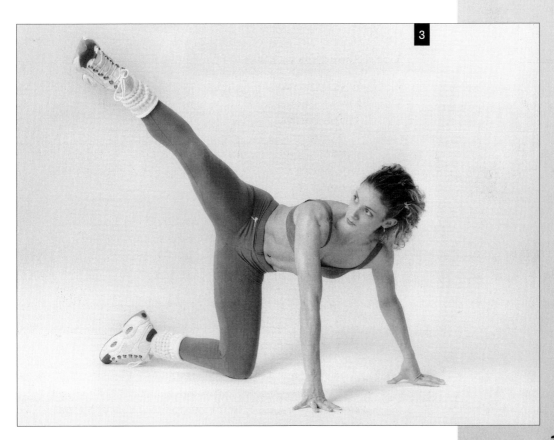

SIDE KICK

Left Side Kick

1 Position yourself on all fours, making sure that your hands, elbows, stomach, and knees are correctly placed as described above.

2 With your left foot flexed, raise your left leg directly to the side so your left thigh is parallel to the floor, or as high as you can raise it comfortably.

3 Execute a Side Kick, stopping two to three inches short of full extension.

4 Immediately recover your leg, bending at the knee while keeping your thigh parallel to the floor, and then lower it to the floor, back to the start position. If you're doing reps, try not to let your left knee touch down. Repeat for two to three sets of 8 reps.

Right Side Kick

1 Position yourself on all fours, making sure that your hands, elbows, stomach, and knees are correctly placed as described above.

2 With your right foot flexed, raise your right leg directly to the side so your right thigh is parallel to the floor, or as high as you can raise it comfortably.

3 Execute a Side Kick, stopping two to three inches short of full extension.

4 Immediately recover your leg, bending at the knee while keeping your thigh parallel to the floor, and then lower it to the floor, back to the start position. If you're doing reps, try not to let your right knee touch down. Repeat for two to three sets of 8 reps.

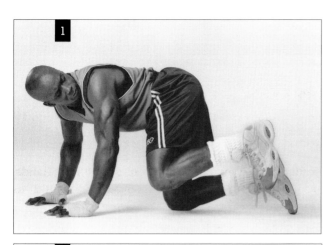

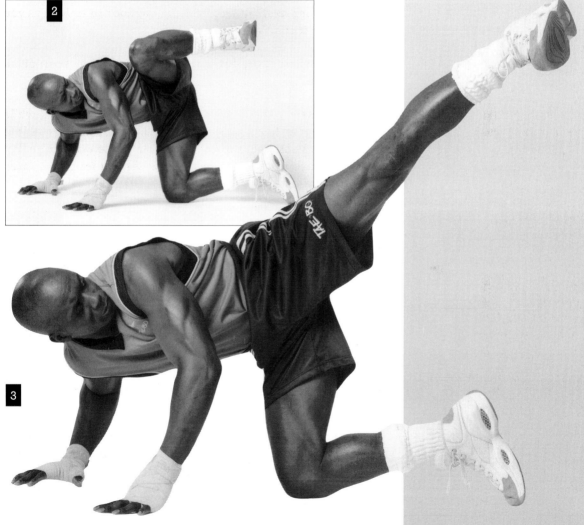

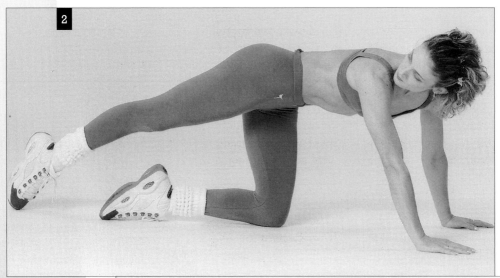

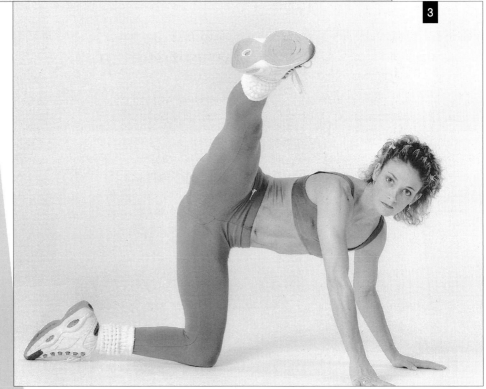

Right Toe Touch/Leg Lift

1. Position yourself on all fours, making sure that your hands, elbows, stomach, and knees are correctly placed as described above.

2. Straighten your right leg directly behind you, two or three inches short of full extension, with your right toes pointed and lightly resting on the floor.

3. Imagine that your right foot is a clock hand that's going backward, from 6:00 to 3:00. (Your head is 12:00.) Focus on contracting your abdominal muscles. Raise your leg as high as you comfortably can. Pull it diagonally toward your shoulder. If you can, work toward raising your foot so it's a couple of inches in front of your shoulder.

4. In a steady, controlled motion, return your right foot to the start position, touching down lightly. Do not let your foot drop or your weight shift over to your right leg. Repeat for two to three sets of 8 reps.

Left Toe Touch/Leg Lift

1. Position yourself on all fours, making sure that your hands, elbows, stomach, and knees are correctly placed as described above.

2. Straighten your left leg directly behind you, two or three inches short of full extension, with your left toes pointed and lightly resting on the floor.

3. Imagine that your left foot is a clock hand that's going forward, from 6:00 to 9:00. (Your head is 12:00.) Focus on contracting your abdominal muscles. Raise your leg as high as you comfortably can. Pull it diagonally toward your shoulder. If you can, work toward raising your foot so it's a couple of inches in front of your shoulder.

4. In a steady, controlled motion, return your left foot to the start position, touching down lightly. Do not let your foot drop or your weight shift over to your left leg. Repeat for two to three sets of 8 reps.

STANDING CRUNCHES

There are two versions of this exercise. Even though the difference between them seems small—the addition of a Knee Raise—they each work a little differently, so the effect is a total ab workout. Every exhalation or crunch counts as "one."

1 Start from a Forward Stance. With your arms at shoulder level and your elbows bent, lightly clasp your hands behind your head. Be sure you're not pulling on your neck as you contract your abdominal muscles. Keep your chest open and your rib cage high.

2 As you exhale to push out all the air, contract your pecs to bring your elbows about halfway in toward the center of your chest, and contract your abdominal muscles to tilt your pelvis upward and bring your upper torso down 10 to 15 degrees. The trick here is to isolate your abdominals so they are the muscles pulling your pelvis up. You shouldn't make this happen by tightening your glutes or your hip flexors.

3 Hold this for a count of 8.

4 Return to the start position, inhale, and repeat for two to three sets of 8 reps.

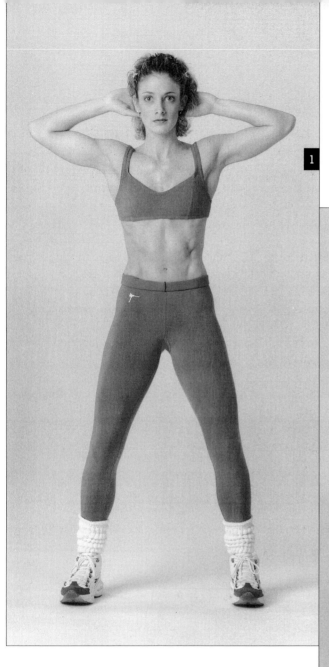

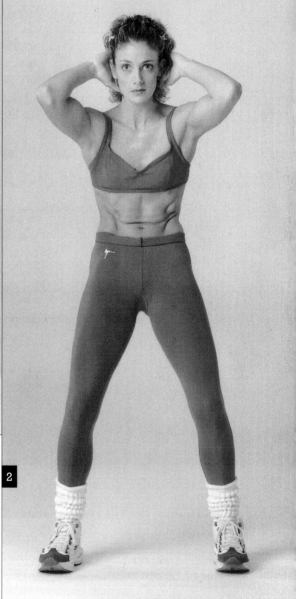

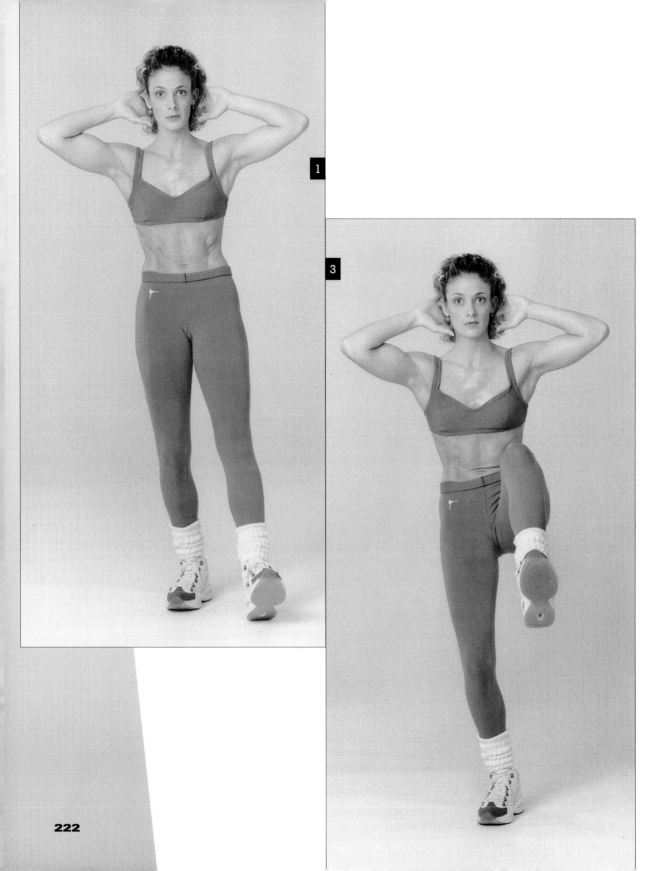

1

3

STANDING CRUNCH WITH KNEE RAISE

1 Start from a Forward Stance. With your arms at shoulder level and your elbows bent, lightly clasp your hands behind your head. Be sure you're not pulling on your neck as you contract your abdominal muscles. Keep your chest open and your rib cage high.

2 As you exhale to push out all the air, contract your pecs to bring your elbows about halfway in toward the center of your chest as you contract your abdominal muscles to tilt your pelvis upward and bring your upper torso down 10 to 15 degrees. The trick here is to isolate your abdominals so they are the muscles pulling your pelvis up. You shouldn't make this happen by tightening your glutes or your hip flexors.

3 As you contract your abs, flex your left foot, shift about 80 percent of your weight to your slightly bent right leg, and contract your abdominal muscles again. As you do, raise your left knee up toward your belly button. As you raise your knee, be careful not to bend forward. Remember: You're bringing your knee to your stomach, not your stomach to your knee.

4 Return to the start position, inhale, and repeat for two to three sets of 8 reps.

5 Repeat with your right knee for two to three sets of 8 reps.

ABDOMINAL CRUNCH WITH KNEE PULL-DOWN

This is a more difficult crunch. It forces you to move slowly and deliberately, so you really work the abs.

1 Lie on your back with your elbows bent and your hands clasped lightly behind your head. Be sure that you're lying with your entire back pressed flat against the floor. Do not arch your back.

2 Raise your legs so your feet are up in the air and your knees are slightly bent. Be sure that your thighs are at a 90-degree angle to your stomach and your knees are in line with your hips.

3 Inhale naturally, and as you exhale, focus on pushing all the air out of your abdomen and contracting your abdominal muscles to pull your knees in toward your stomach. At the same time, raise your head and upper chest toward your knees. Press your elbows together without using your arms to pull your neck forward.

4 Return to the start position and repeat for two to three sets of 8 reps.

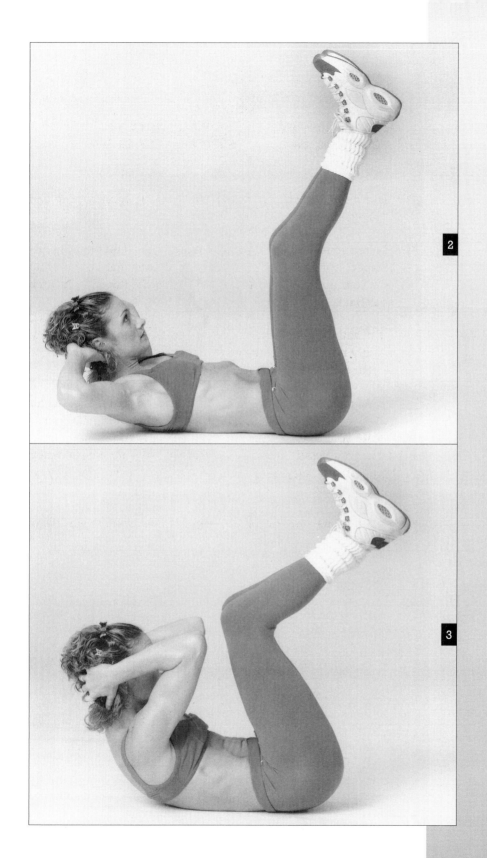

2

3

225

OBLIQUE CRUNCH

This is an advanced, challenging movement. If this is not comfortable, then just concentrate on moving one leg, your upper (in this case, your left) leg. If you can do only one or two reps, that's okay. Regular ab work doesn't always work the muscles at your sides, the obliques. This is a great exercise for firming the abductors and the obliques and helping define your waistline. If you're not really feeling this along your sides, you're not working the right muscles.

1 Lie on your right side with your knees and feet together and stretched out straight, a few inches above the floor and parallel to the ceiling. Extend your right arm on the floor with your palm down against the floor. Rise up on your right elbow. Your left arm is bent and your left hand is resting behind your head.

2 With your left hand resting behind your head, contract your abdominal muscles and exhale. At the same time, raise both legs off the floor as high as you comfortably can. Be sure to bend both at the knee, and pull your knees toward your stomach with your abdominal muscles, not your legs.

3 Release and return to start position. This should be a very controlled movement; do not let your legs fall back down. Repeat for two to three sets of 8 reps.

4 Repeat on your left side for two to three sets of 8 reps.

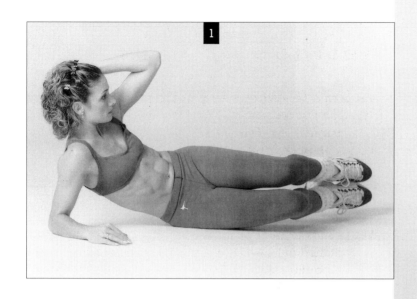

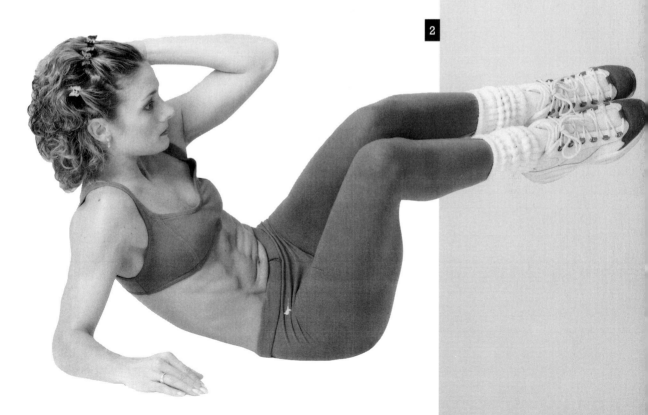

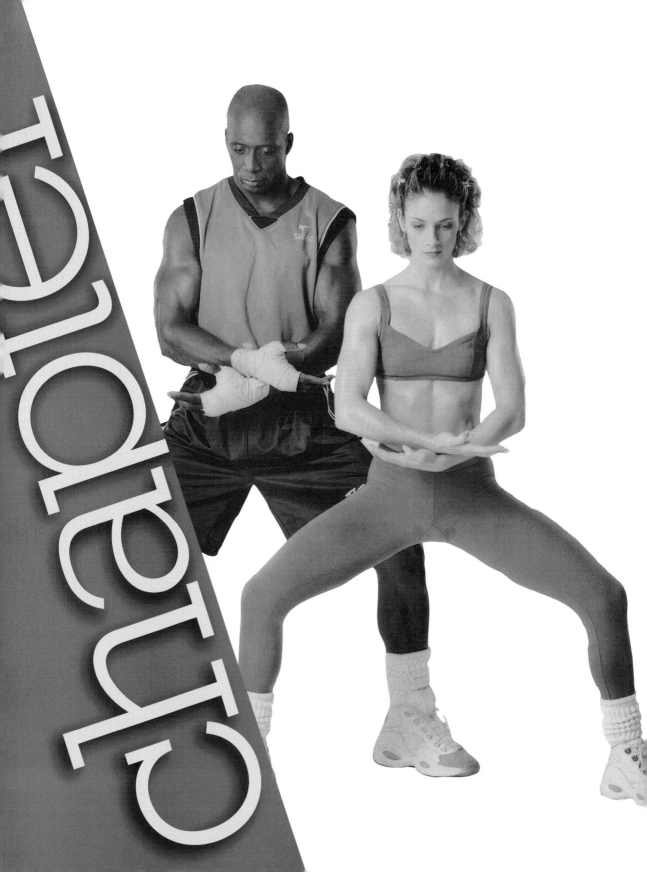

eleven

The Cooldown

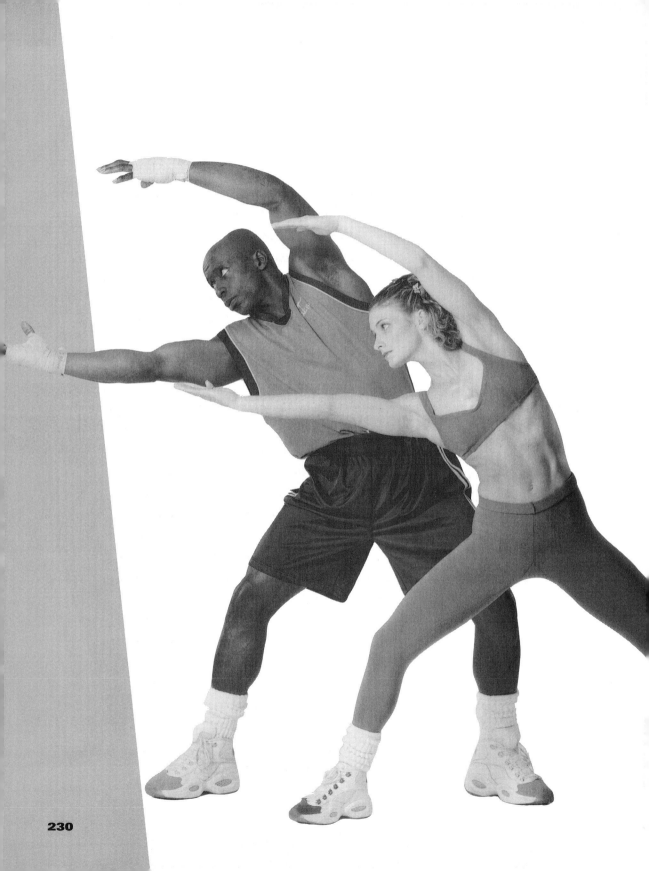

Cooldown

You've worked hard and done a great job! I'll bet you feel stronger and ready for anything. Now it's time to do the Cooldown. Remember: Never skip the Cooldown. Even if you're so busy that you feel you need to cut five minutes off your Workout, take it out of the middle—never the Warm-up or the Cooldown.

Your body needs to cool down—and gradually slow down—to give your heart, your lungs, and your muscles a chance to recover and return to their natural, resting states. After any intense physical activity, your body begins a natural slowing-down process. If you stop moving abruptly, you run the risk of a sudden drop in blood pressure (and possibly fainting), as well as increased muscle soreness and tightness.

Before you begin the Cooldown, it's essential that you spend about five minutes walking around the room or marching in place. When you do this, you're helping your heart cool down, because your leg muscles are actually acting as pumps to return blood from your legs to your heart. When you don't include walking or marching in your pre-Cooldown routine, your heart has to work too hard.

Your Cooldown can also tell you something about your fitness level. The better your fitness level, the more quickly your body will return to its natural state. If it takes you longer than ten minutes to bring your heart rate and your breathing back to normal, you may be working out at a level that's too challenging for your current level of fitness. You've worked too hard to walk off the floor not feeling your best.

As you become more comfortable with the Cooldown, it should become as fluid as a dance. Be aware of each movement and breathe naturally throughout. Through it all, you should feel totally relaxed. Visualize creating a peaceful circle of air around you. As you become more familiar with the Cooldown, try closing your eyes as you move. Let yourself flow into it.

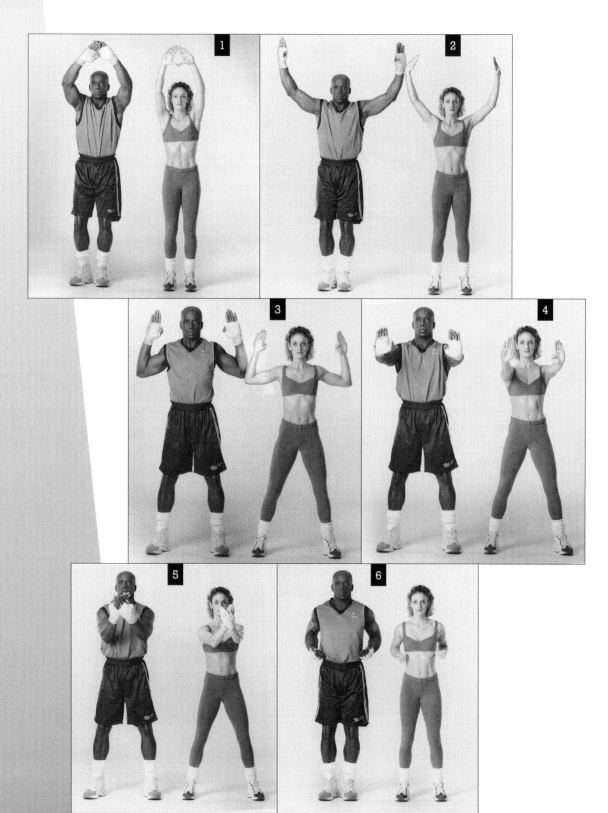

THE COOLDOWN

1 Stand naturally, facing forward, with your feet parallel and about hip-distance apart. Your knees should be slightly bent and your arms should be relaxed, in front of your body, with your hands crossed loosely at the wrists. Extend your arms out to your sides, and lift them up over your head until you are lightly touching your fingers together.

2 With your palms open and facing forward, slowly start bringing your arms down.

3 Stop when your hands are parallel to your ears and your elbows are bent.

4 Push forward with both arms as if you're pushing something away from you or creating that peaceful circle of air. As you push, exhale.

5 With your arms still fully extended, turn your palms so they face you and loosely cross your hands.

6 Make a fist with each hand and pull your fists toward you, so you end with your elbows bent, arms against your rib cage, and your fists upturned.

7 Flip your fists so your palms are facing downward, open your hands, and push toward the floor. As you do this, remember that you want to stand straight and stretch your arms and keep your shoulders level.

8 Slowly bend forward and continue pushing down. As you bend your knees, be sure that they're not extending beyond your toes.

9 Slowly rise to standing, turning your hands so your palms are facing upward and are loosely crossed at the wrists.

10 As you imagine tracing a circle around you, stretch your arms downward and then up until they're at your sides and your fingers are just a little higher than your head. Your palms should be facing outward.

11 In one count, in a sweeping, controlled motion, step out into a Horse Stance while bringing your arms down in front of you. Again, your wrists are loosely crossed.

12 Bring your hands directly over your head, fully extending your arms with your palms facing inward. Stretch over to your left. Concentrate on stretching rather than bending at the waist. Hold for a count of 8.

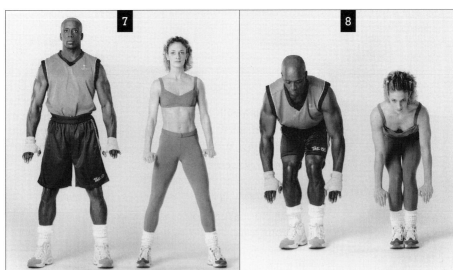

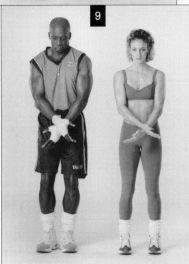

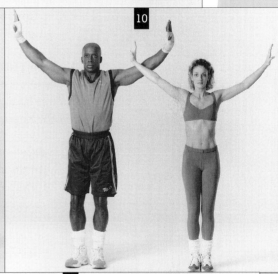

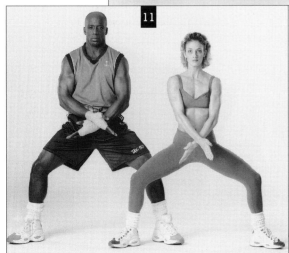

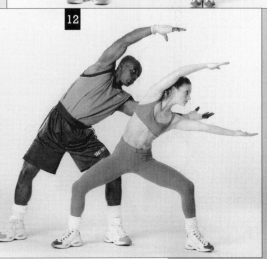

235

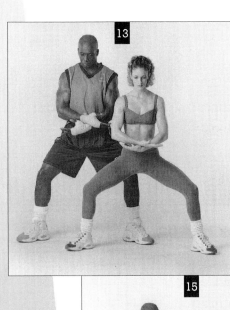

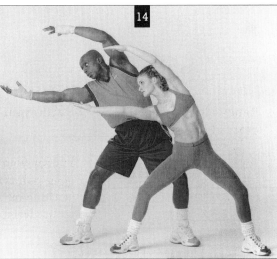

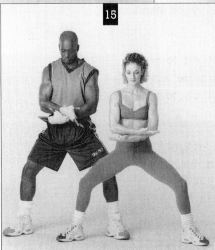

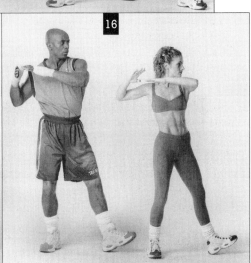

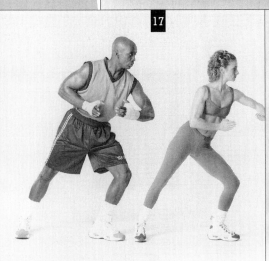

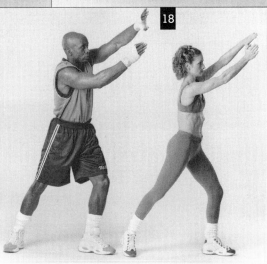

13 Return to the Horse Stance, with your hands crossed in front of you.

14 Again bring your hands directly over your head, fully extending your arms with your palms facing inward. Stretch over to your right. Concentrate on stretching rather than bending at the waist. Hold for a count of 8.

15 Return to the Horse Stance, with your hands crossed in front of you.

16 Looking to the left, shift your weight to your right leg. Pivot on your left heel to the left as you raise your arms, bent at the elbow, toward your right shoulder.

17 Drop your left toes and shift your weight forward as you bring your bent arms down toward your waist. Stretch over your left leg without bending at the waist.

18 Still facing left, raise your hands above your head, about shoulder-distance apart, with your elbows slightly bent.

19 Pivot through the motion, following your arms.

20 You'll find yourself facing right in the same position.

21 Looking to the right, shift your weight to your left leg. Pivot on your right heel to the right as you raise your arms, bent at the elbow, toward your left shoulder.

22 Drop your right toes and shift your weight forward as you bring your bent arms down toward your waist. Stretch over your right leg without bending at the waist.

23 Still facing right, raise your hands above your head, about shoulder-distance apart, with your elbows slightly bent.

24 As you face forward, shift your weight to your bent right leg so you're only touching down lightly with your left toe. At the same time, bring your extended arms down until they're about parallel with your hips.

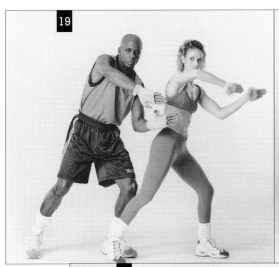

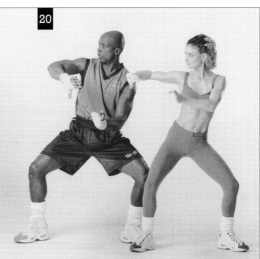

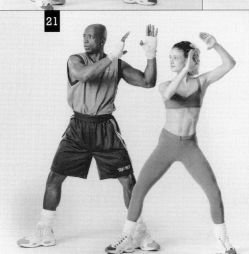

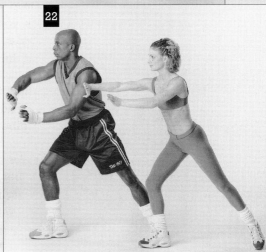

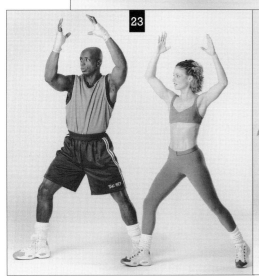

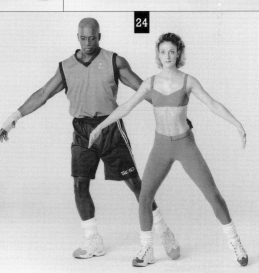

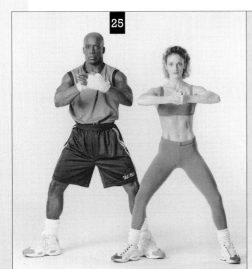

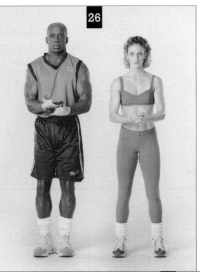

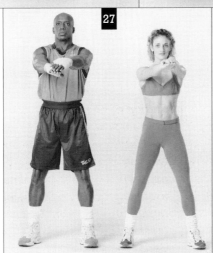

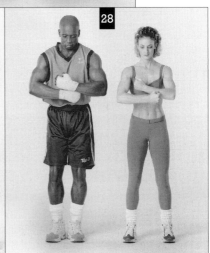

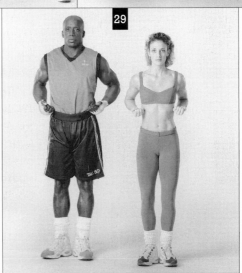

25 Step back into the Horse Stance. Bend your elbows and clasp your hands in front of your chest. Your arms will be parallel to the floor, just a few inches lower than your shoulder.

26 Keeping your hands clasped together, bring them down to your belly button.

27 Then extend your arms forward, straight in front of you.

28 Bring your arms back toward your body, form fists, and place your left forearm a few inches above and parallel to your right forearm.

29 Rotate your fists so your palms face upward and pull both back toward your waist. Holding that position, bend forward at the hips, keeping your back level and your knees slightly bent.

30 Bow.

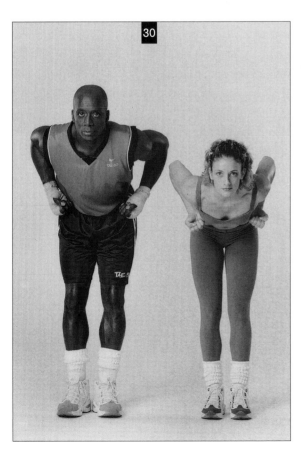

Ending with a bow is a tradition from martial arts that I've carried into Tae-Bo, because it's a way of marking completion, expressing respect to those around you, and showing humbleness toward your teacher and the work you've dedicated yourself to. As you bow, take a few moments to think about these things before the everyday world rushes back in.

How do you feel? Great, I'll bet. And you deserve to. Now take this feeling with you through the rest of your day, and be a conqueror in everything you do. That's the Tae-Bo Way.

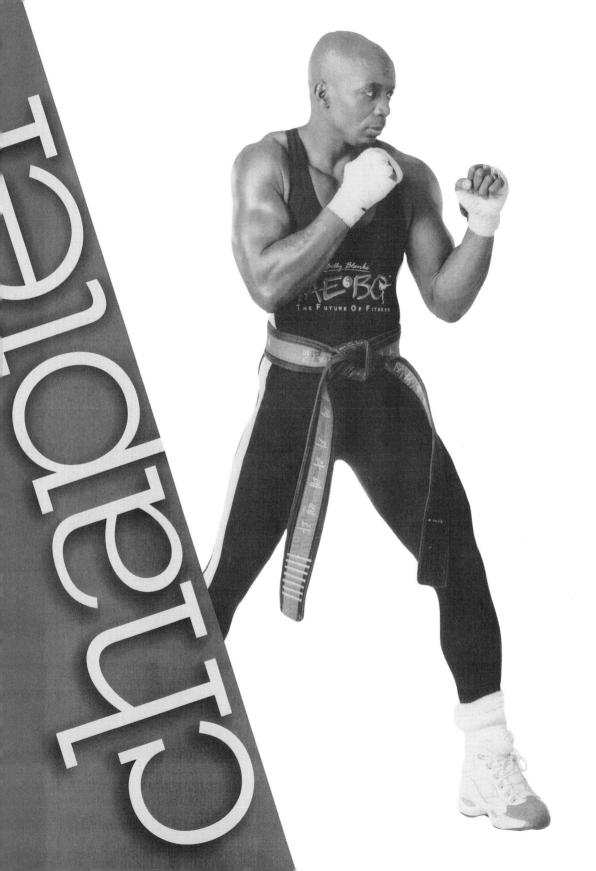

twelve

Making Tae-Bo
Last a Lifetime

I hope that you've enjoyed reading—and working out with—*The Tae-Bo Way,* the most complete guide to Tae-Bo. It's everything you need to know, but it's not everything that there is to know—and that's an important difference. There are many more things that you can learn from Tae-Bo, but I can't tell you exactly what they are, because from now on, you are the teacher. I said before, If you have the will, I have the way. Now, you have to make it *your* way.

If you're like most of my students, just doing Tae-Bo has changed you, both outside and in. I'm happy when students tell me about the lost pounds and inches, how great they feel and how much better they think they look. And don't misunderstand me: Those are great goals to work toward. I hope that you have also felt a change inside. If you have more confidence, more strength, more focus, and more desire to go even farther, then Tae-Bo has exercised more than your body. It has exercised and strengthened your will. If Tae-Bo has taught you to do just one thing you never thought you could do before, you've learned something valuable about yourself. You've learned that the power to change lies within yourself. You've learned that you are your own boss, your own teacher, your own protector, your own person in every way. You are a conqueror.

At the beginning, when these experiences are new and fresh, it's easy to keep up your enthusiasm. But how do you keep it going next year and the year after that? I have students who have been doing Tae-Bo for over a decade, and there is a way to keep the challenges and the rewards alive for you too. Even though I developed Tae-Bo and have done these exercises more than a million times over the years, I'm still learning. I want people to look at me and see the real Billy Blanks. Take away the titles and the accomplishments, and in the end you have the man I face in the mirror every morning at five A.M. before I go to the gym: just a man who works hard at what he believes in. Just a man who saw his own life transformed and wants to share what he's learned with others.

Tae-Bo is about learning, about letting old ideas you may have had about yourself, your body, your will, and your spirit fall away. It's about letting new ideas come in, and then doing the work to make them part of your life. It's about reaching that point where your body falls under the power of your spirit and your will. It's about working toward goals that don't show up in the mirror but are reflected in everything you do. It's about using your body to reach a new understanding of who you are inside, your spirit.

Keeping Your Tae-Bo Workout Fresh

There's no end to Tae-Bo, no number of reps or combination of moves you can master and consider yourself "done." There are countless ways to keep your Workout fresh and challenging. You can keep adding to your Tae-Bo videotape library, so you have variety in your Workouts. You can mix up your videotapes too. Instead of doing one Workout all the way through, you can randomly fast-forward through a few different Tae-Bo Workout tapes and do half of one videotape and then switch to a second tape for the second half. You may reach a point with your Workout where you do it without looking at the screen, and just listen to the instructions. Or you can do your Workout by watching the videotape with the sound off. Or you can try doing at least one set of every exercise with your eyes closed. Each way challenges different senses and different skills.

Also have your mental guard up for those moments when you start to feel that it's all coming a little too easily for you. It's important to recognize the difference between a Workout where you've got the technique and timing down so tight, it just flows, and a Workout that kicks quickly into automatic and leaves you not doing much except going through the motions. Either of these can be a solid aerobic workout, but if there's nothing going on between you and your Workout, something's bound to happen. You're either going to hurt yourself because you're no longer as keenly aware of what your body is doing, or you're going to get bored and quit.

You can always—and you should always—stop the videotape whenever you need extra time to master a technique or smooth out a combination. You can also pause to add one, two, or three additional sets of an exercise. If certain moves seem beyond you now, try working on them outside your Workout. One student I know who often works late at her desk does ten minutes of combinations to Stevie Wonder to get her energy up and improve that part of her Workout. You can practice balancing on one leg (with your knee slightly bent, of course) or improving your Horse Stance when you're talking on the phone or watching television. You can practice just being more keenly aware of your own body and everything around you.

One way to keep your Workout interesting is to end each with a goal for the next one. While it's still fresh in your mind, think about what you did well and what came easily. Then think about the rough spots still ahead. Choose one move or technique and promise yourself you'll work on it next time. Also remember that no matter how easy or difficult a particular Workout is for you, you gained something. Tae-Bo works on so many different levels, no Workout is ever a total loss. You might be tired or under the weather when you work out. But the important thing is that you still came to work out. Maybe you can't get those knee raises up as high as you usually do, or your punches just don't have that snap you expect. Don't be discouraged. Accept that maybe today's Workout won't be the best you've ever done, but don't overlook what else is getting a Workout of a different kind: your patience, your dedication, your ability to be clear and honest about your performance. Or your body might be giving one hundred percent while personal problems are making it difficult for your mind to completely focus. At the very least, you've gotten a good aerobic workout. Remember: Just having the commitment to stick with something when you know you're not doing as well as you could is quite an accomplishment. This is the time when a lot of people would quit. Instead, you've used your will to take control when your body or your mind wasn't up to the job. That in itself should inspire you to work harder next time.

Tae-Bo Is for Any Time

It's never too late to start Tae-Bo, and never too early, either. One of the best things to come out of Tae-Bo for me personally was the experience of having my whole family working out together. Our children today are the least fit generation in history. I find it discouraging to see how many mothers and fathers wait in line, sometimes for more than an hour, to get inside the Billy Blanks World Karate Center to do their Tae-Bo, while at home their kids are watching television or playing video games. Everyone understands the health risks these kids face now and may face as they grow older. It's a serious problem that deserves a lot more attention than it's getting. We all focus on the negative physical effects of this non-active lifestyle, but what about the spiritual side of it? What about how much happiness and satisfaction kids today miss because they don't challenge themselves physically and never get the chance to find their will, let alone build it?

I think Tae-Bo is a great family activity, for many reasons. It's a good way for families to spend time together and get to know one another on a new level. When you're working out, especially with something that's as physically, mentally, and spiritually challenging as Tae-Bo, you may show your children sides of your personality they've never seen before. Face it, unless your child spends every minute with you each day, he probably has no idea what your workday is like. If you're like many parents, you've seen to it that your child doesn't witness you struggling or attempting something you've never done before. Being a parent myself, I know it's important to be the boss when it comes to kids. But that doesn't mean that you're always the expert. Sometimes you can learn from your children, and I can't imagine anything that can make a child feel more powerful or give him a greater sense of self-esteem than to know that he has the power to help his own parent. I know from my own experience, there's something awesome about hearing your own child encouraging you to keep going or offering you advice on your technique. And as a parent, I know that by seeing my wife and me work so hard, my children have a different kind of respect for us. No amount of talking could ever communicate to your child the importance of will and determination, as well as him seeing you put those values into practice. Children learn more from what we do than from what we say. Show your children through your example what it means to work hard, to push yourself, and to not give up.

Tae-Bo Is for Every Season

The beauty of Tae-Bo is that no matter where you are in your life—no matter what your age, ability, or physical condition—you can do Tae-Bo. Because always remember: Tae-Bo works from the inside out. It works with you, by offering you ways to work around or through those parts that may be difficult for you today. All I have taught you about Tae-Bo—every move, every combination, every technique—can be modified so you can do it.

There's also no beginning to Tae-Bo and no end. As long as you're doing your Workout, as long as you're giving it your best and pushing yourself to the next level, you're making real progress. Tae-Bo doesn't ask you to compare yourself to anyone else, only to yourself. Are you in some way, no matter how small, better than you were the day before? If you can't do even one more kick than you did yesterday, do you at least believe that you will tomorrow or the day after? Do you at least have the faith in yourself to know that you will work at it? Do you have the focus and the will to work toward that goal? If you do, then you have made progress, even if it's the kind that no one can see with their eyes. Think how much better every aspect of your life can be if you just apply that positive, determined attitude.

Your Tae-Bo Way

Since Tae-Bo has taken off in the past year, I've been asked hundreds of times, "What is it about Tae-Bo that makes people stick with it? Why are they so excited? Why are they so dedicated? Why has Tae-Bo grown?" I like to think that it isn't Tae-Bo that's grown as much as it is all the people who have let themselves grow through Tae-Bo. With Tae-Bo, everyone who works hard gets what they came for in the first place—the physical change—and then they realize they're also getting something else. That something else is a new attitude, a self-confidence, a way of looking at stones in your pathway and immediately saying not "I will try . . ." but "I will." It's the "something" that I felt as a young boy in karate when I discovered the connection between my body, my mind, and my spirit. It was the power to tap in to my will and start believing in what I could do. It was the power to listen to my own body, my own thoughts, my own spirit, and to hear what they told me. I learned to believe in that, not in what others were saying about who I was and what I could do. Those were their thoughts, not my own.

Now you are the teacher. I hope that *The Tae-Bo Way* will help you find your own way.

Acknowledgments

First and foremost, I would like to give all the glory to God. He gave his only begotten son that I might be saved. Lord, I am very honored and privileged to be used as a vessel, to help give life to people through Tae-Bo. I thank you for the receptive hearts that have embraced this total Workout. I appreciate all your blessings; to whom much is given, of him much is expected.

Lord Jesus Christ, I strive to continually let my light shine for the glory of your kingdom, seeking you first. Through your Word I have come to know that all things are possible, for I walk by faith, not by sight.

To everyone who has made Tae-Bo a way of life, I sincerely thank you for testing your spirit, mind, and body. Now you know that you are the one in control. I am merely a guide, but you put forth the effort. You have exercised your free will. I feel truly blessed when one person tells me that Tae-Bo has changed his life for the better. That is what it's all about.

I would like to acknowledge my wife, Gayle, for giving me the opportunity to be the best I can be in everything I do, for sticking by my side through trials and tribulations, and for always being faithful to God's Word. I thank her for being my best friend, my lover, the mother of our children, and my spinal cord. Without her, none of this would be possible. God bless her and keep her strong in health. I love you so much.

To my children, Shellie and Billy Jr., you are the lights of my life. I am proud to be your dad. I love you both with all my heart, and I want to see you always have good days. Remember, God is good, keep your eyes on him.

Shellie, you are my sidekick and you are definitely Daddy's girl. I'm so very proud of the beautiful young woman you have become, inside and out. Your lovely spirit shines. Thank you for your help and hard work in bringing this book to life.

Billy Jr., I'm proud that you are my son. Your heart is so much like mine, always remember that. You are a multitalented person with so much to offer. Break out and shine on. You are more than a conqueror.

To all of my family, thank you for your love and support over the years. You are all special to me, I love you.

To Betty, I love you, you are in a better place. To Michael, Irene, Winnie, Raymond, Charles, Thelma, David, Marie, John, Kenny, Stevie, Willie, and Joe, God bless you all.

To my mother-in-law, Mrs. Janet Godfrey, I love you. Thank you for giving me your daughter, the key to my life. You have always and unfailingly supported me throughout the years. Thank you for believing in me and my dreams when others were laughing and ridiculing. I will never forget it.

To the rest of my wife's family—Bob, Nadene, and Paul Godfrey—thank you for your support over the years.

To my pastor, Frederick K. C. Price, you are my teacher and mentor. You truly are a man of integrity and honor. Thank you for being so bold, for speaking the truth and never compromising. Your teachings have helped open my heart to the Gospel. You taught me that it was a guide for life, now, in this present day. Through the Word you have shown me what my rights and privileges are, why Jesus died for me. Therefore you have been instrumental in changing my life and my family's life. I extend my sincerest gratitude to you.

To Dr. Betty Price, you are such a sweet and special woman of God, one of grace and peace. Thank you for being a part of my family's life. To the rest of the Price family—Angie and Michael Evans, Cheryl and Allen Crabbe, Stephanie and Danon Buchanan, and Frederick Price Jr.—you are all very special people, and my wife and I thank God for you.

To my brothers and sisters in Christ at Crenshaw Christian Center, we are of one blood. I love you all in the name of Jesus.

To Patty Romanowski, I sincerely appreciate everything you have done in bringing the Tae-Bo Way to text. Your work over the past several months reflects your caring, dignified, and professional manner. Thank you for really listening to me, for being open-minded and receptive, and most of all for capturing my spirit on paper. I have faith that your efforts will help touch the hearts and lives of many.

To everyone at Bantam Books, particularly Irwyn Applebaum, Nita Taublib, Robin Michaelson, Jim Plumeri, Glen Edelstein, Kelly Chian, Maggie Hart, and Amanda Kavanagh, thank you for all your support and guidance. You have blessed me with an amazing opportunity to help people be more fit physically and spiritually.

I also appreciate the insight of Neil Sol, Ph.D.

To Paul Monet, words cannot adequately express my appreciation to you. We have forged a great friendship and a mutual sense of respect for one another. Together we have had a vision of changing one life at a time. I thank God that you had the foresight and faith in me and Tae-Bo to bring it to the world. Thank you for letting me speak the truth from my heart. Thank you for never asking me to compromise in any way; I greatly respect you for that. We have set a new standard, and we have let people know that they are empowered by their own spirit. If they have the will, Tae-Bo is the way.

To Mark Amuso, thank you for your extraordinary hard work on the infomercial and all the tapes. You have tirelessly striven to present Tae-Bo in a first-class format. I appreciate your allowing me to be myself. I appreciate your support and your friendship.

To everyone else at NCP Marketing—Paul Monet Jr., Michelle Reber, Gene Boyer, Dave Simmons, Colleen Jones, and all the crew—you have blessed my life. Thank you.

To my manager, Jeffrey Greenfield, thank you for your guidance and advice, and above all, thank you for your friendship. You are a dear friend to me and my family and that is the most important aspect of our relationship. We have witnessed amazing blessings together; what a testimony to faith and hard work. God bless you, your lovely wife, Shelly, and your dear daughter, Yosepha, always.

To Jan Yoss, my counselor, my friend. Your integrity and moral character are without question. You are my advocate on so many levels. I appreciate your honesty and your brilliance, but also your loving-kindness. The special friendship that Gayle and I share with you is extremely special to us. Thank you and God bless.

To John Younesi, thank you for helping to pull things together. Your effort is sincerely appreciated. I look forward to the future, knowing that you and Jan have my best interests at heart. God bless you and yours.

To Dave Paller, thank you for your advice in many areas of my life. Most of all I appreciate your work with the Billy Blanks Foundation, which Gayle and I are so excited about. We look forward to having an impact on women's and children's issues. God bless you.

Julieanne Hartman, thank you for assisting me in so many ways. You are a special friend. Your fun personality has made working with you a joy. God bless you, Butchie, Carly, and Sophia.

John Arthur, thank you for keeping an eye out for me and for just plain being a friend. Friends are hard to find.

Trevor Ziemba, you've got my back, and I appreciate it. You have become a special friend and buddy. Thanks for looking out for me and mine. Love in Christ.

To Lenny Walters, my friend in Christ. God bless you, brother.

To Walt Gorsey, thank you for all your effort during the past several months. I appreciate your representing me with integrity.

To Barry Fields, I thank you for helping to shape the graphic image and branding of the Tae-Bo Way. Your hard work and effort have not gone unnoticed.

To John Hileman, thank you for keeping my affairs in order. Gayle and I appreciate your loyalty, hard work, and dedication. God bless you.

To JoBee Croskery and her crew, thank you for your ability to photographically capture my spirit and essence. What a pleasure it has been working with you all. JoBee, God bless you, you are so sweet.

A special thanks to the graphic design firm of Gillis & Smiler for their creativity in helping to develop a brand image for Tae-Bo and Billy Blanks Enterprises.

To Judy Biore, thanks for being a friend and a loyal supporter over the years.

To Magic Johnson and Magic Johnson Productions, thank you for taking Tae-Bo live throughout the United States. What a great experience. God bless you all.

To the people of Erie, Pennsylvania, my hometown, thank you for your support over the years.

To my entire staff at the Billy Blanks World Training Center in Sherman Oaks, California, and Billy Blanks Enterprises, thank you for your hard work, support, and loyalty. Bringing Tae-Bo to the world is an incredible blessing. Thank you for the roles you have played in this endeavor; I appreciate your dedication and my sincere gratitude is extended to you all. You know what place you each hold in my heart. God bless each and every one of you.

An important expression of thanks is owed to my core Tae-Bo family at the Billy Blanks World Training Center, those of you who have been with me from the beginning. You know who you are. Thank you for loving Tae-Bo and for staying loyal through the many transitions. Yes, it's grown. As my manager said, "We invited one hundred and twenty people to a party and one thousand showed up." What a blessing. I appreciate your unselfishness and want to thank you for allowing me to share Tae-Bo with the world. Lives have been changed. Isn't that awesome?

Finally, to all martial-arts practioners throughout the world, karate is my foundation, my true love.

About the Author

Billy Blanks is the creator of Tae-Bo, the revolutionary fitness program that blends elements of martial arts, boxing, and dance. His *Tae-Bo Workout* videotapes are the top-selling exercise series in history. Based on Billy's philosophy that true physical fitness must involve and inspire the mind and the spirit, Tae-Bo proves that, as Billy says, "Physical fitness is about more than the physical. It's about exercising your will to change yourself from the inside. Once you change yourself on the inside, the outside will fall into place."

Billy is the fourth of fifteen children born to Isaac and Mabeline Blanks in Erie, Pennsylvania. Growing up amid poverty and hampered by undiagnosed dyslexia and a hip-tendon anomaly, Billy was physically awkward, quiet, and shy. He credits discovering karate at age twelve with changing his life. At sixteen, he received his first black belt. Billy holds a seventh-degree black belt in tae kwon do, in addition to black belts in five other

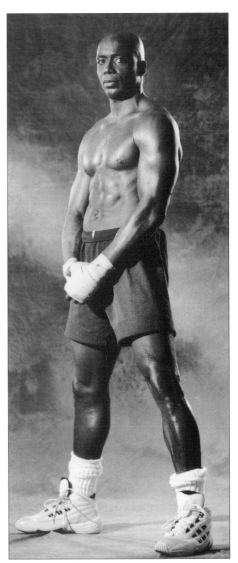

martial arts. He has earned numerous awards in international karate competitions, including seven world championships, and he was captain of the U.S. Karate Team in 1980. Billy has been in the Karate Hall of Fame since 1982 and has also earned two Golden Gloves titles for boxing. He has traveled the world competing and teaching, and has received many awards, including the South African Humanitarian Award for Outstanding Sportsmanship in 1978.

In 1989, he established the Billy Blanks World Karate Center in Sherman Oaks, California, the home of Tae-Bo. Billy has personally trained hundreds of people from every walk of life, from professional athletes and movie stars to physically challenged people. In addition to teaching and training, Billy has acted in dozens of movies, including *Kiss the Girls* and *The Last Boy Scout*, and has appeared on dozens of television programs, including a cameo on *ER*. With his wife, Gayle, he heads the Billy Blanks Foundation, a philanthropic organization established to aid a variety of causes that benefit women and children.

Billy and Gayle have two children, Shellie and Billy Jr. They make their home in southern California.

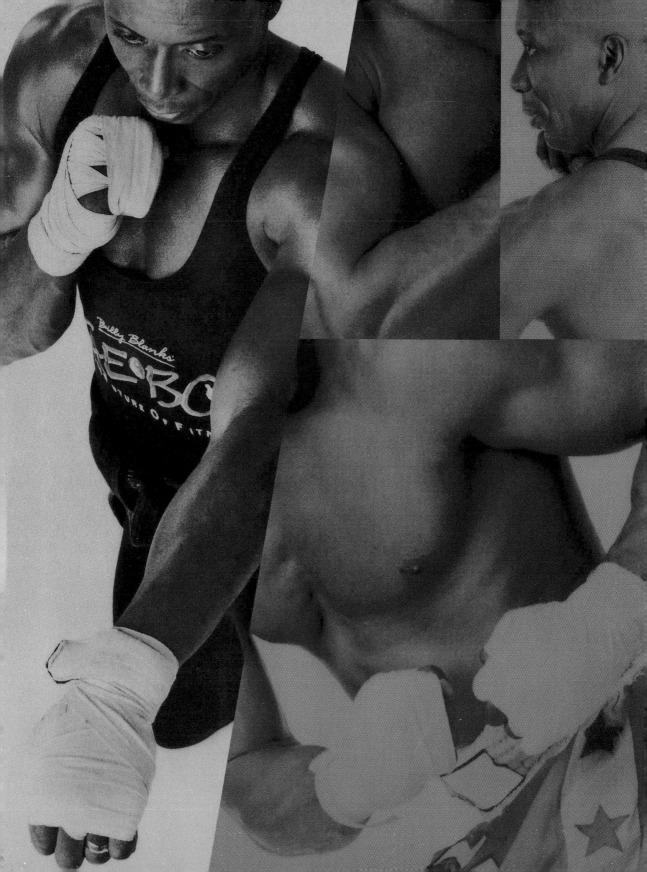